Imaging of Plastic Surgery of the Breast and Other Implants

Stéphanie Cohen-Zarade

Imaging of Plastic Surgery of the Breast and Other Implants

A Practical Approach

Springer

Stéphanie Cohen-Zarade
Institut de Radiologie de Paris
Paris, France

ISBN 978-3-031-64158-9 ISBN 978-3-031-64159-6 (eBook)
https://doi.org/10.1007/978-3-031-64159-6

The original submitted manuscript has been translated into English. The translation was done using artificial intelligence. A subsequent revision was performed by the author(s) to further refine the work and to ensure that the translation is appropriate concerning content and scientific correctness. It may, however, read stylistically different from a conventional translation.

Translation from the French language edition: “Imagerie en Chirurgie Esthétique Mammaire et Autres Implants” by Stéphanie Cohen-Zarade, © Sauramps Medical 2022. Published by Sauramps Medical. All Rights Reserved.

This Springer imprint is published by the registered company Springer Nature Switzerland AG
The registered company address is: Gewerbestrasse 11, 6330 Cham, Switzerland

Foreword

As an ever-evolving field, plastic surgery of the breast demands a specialized approach to diagnostic imaging. The field of breast augmentation has traversed several controversies in the past decades and witnessed remarkable progress, offering women several alternatives, in multiple varied clinical scenarios, to consider for plastic surgery of the breasts to improve their well-being.

Drawing from her experience as a radiologist in a private radiology practice in Paris that specializes in preoperative and post-surgery surveillance of breast and other types of plastic surgeries, Stéphanie Cohen-Zarade navigates the complexities of various imaging modalities for implants in the light of her specialized practice, discussing the complexities and challenges inherent in the imaging of these patients.

This book is extensively illustrated, with radiologic images of all modalities used for breast imaging—mammography, ultrasound, and magnetic resonance imaging—as well as some schematic diagrams that all contribute to appreciating the nuances and subtleties of breast imaging. Each chapter is written to provide an accessible resource, with rich iconography and practical insights based on the author's years of experience. The author's recommendations are often universal, although occasionally, there are particularities that are specific to a practice in France, with screening and surveillance algorithms that may differ from those in other parts of the world.

In addition to breast augmentation with implants and breast reduction and mastopexy, the topics of lipofilling, augmentation through injection of less conventional agents, and male breast surgery are also covered. The last chapter offers a glimpse into imaging of other implants, shedding light on newer dimensions of patient care rarely covered in radiological textbooks.

Dr. Cohen-Zarade's commitment to patient care resonates throughout this work. Her dedication to advancing the understanding of the field of plastic surgery of the breast and imaging of various implants is undeniable, as well as a profound passion for ensuring the highest standards in patient care. This resource provides a practical and richly illustrated guide to equally guide newcomers to the world of breast plastic surgery imaging and seasoned practitioners to improve the care of patients with implants.

Montreal, QC, Canada Isabelle Trop

Preface

Dr. Stéphanie Cohen-Zarade is a specialist in breast imaging and oncology within a large private radiology group. In this context, she also became interested in imaging after cosmetic breast surgery, and the plastic surgeons with whom she collaborates now refer their patients to her for the monitoring of various other surgeries performed (contrast-enhanced abdominal computed tomography before DIEP flap, for example).

This book helps the readers immerse themselves in the images she has been able to collect, which they will encounter even in the context of screening or monitoring of breast cancer.

Paris, France Stéphanie Cohen-Zarade

Contents

About the Author

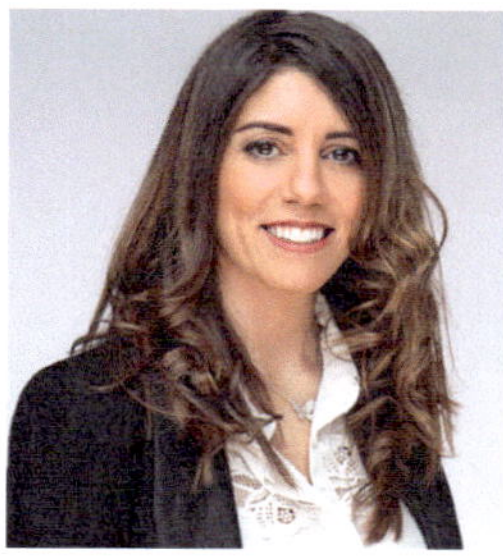

Stéphanie Cohen-Zarade Currently a partner at the "Institut de Radiologie de Paris," specialized in the field of breast imaging, Dr. Stéphanie Cohen-Zarade completed medical school at the University Paris VII. She finished residency in diagnostic and interventional radiology at Institut Curie. She completed a fellowship in breast imaging and interventional imaging at Saint Louis Hospital, where she served as chief fellow. She obtained the university diploma of "breast pathology" at Versailles University, "women's imaging" at Paris VI University, "head and neck imaging" at Paris V University, and the FORCOMED training (organized breast cancer screening in France). She completed the "Clinical Research Training Course" (NIH office of clinical research training and medical education). She is also the author of scientific articles and is writing a monthly publication about breast imaging in the journal *Gynécologie pratique*. She is a member of the French Society of Radiology (SFR) and the French Society of Breast Imaging (SIFEM). She is teaching at Saint Louis Hospital for the university diploma of breast diseases.

General Radioanatomy of the Breast and Imaging Techniques

1

Contents

Breasts play a major role in a woman's self-image and her femininity [1, 2].

Cosmetic breast surgery is one of the most performed procedures in plastic surgery, and it has experienced an unprecedented boom since the early 90s.

However, it is necessary to perform breast imaging both in the context of cancer screening but also to monitor some of the aesthetic interventions performed.

It is therefore important to know what the indications of imaging are for preoperative, postoperative and follow-up, to understand the usual post-surgical aspects, as well as the possible complications.

The different imaging techniques used are mammography (X-rays), tomosynthesis, ultrasound (ultrasound), and the most sensitive technique which is MRI (Magnetic Resonance Imaging). Technological innovations such as artificial intelligence through computer-aided diagnostic (CAD) systems, helps for a better analysis of the glandular structure (Fig. 1.1).

The CT scan, because of its low resolution and radiation dose, is not suitable for breast imaging even though it happens that we incidentally detect breast masses, lymph nodes or an already advanced complication of an implant (Fig. 1.2a, b).

The radiologist specialized in senology must be part of a multidisciplinary approach, with clinical knowledge of breast pathology and the different surgical interventions for aesthetic purposes.

S. Cohen-Zarade, *Imaging of Plastic Surgery of the Breast and Other Implants*,
https://doi.org/10.1007/978-3-031-64159-6_1

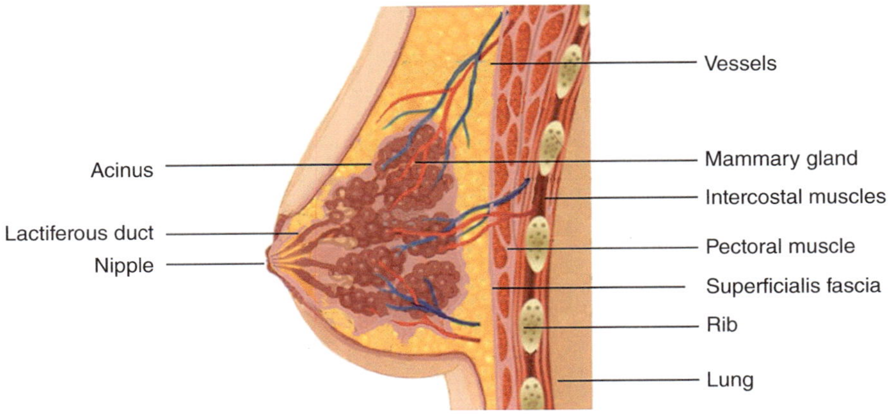

Fig. 1.1 Profile view of a breast. *Drawing by Jean-Charles Goldberg*

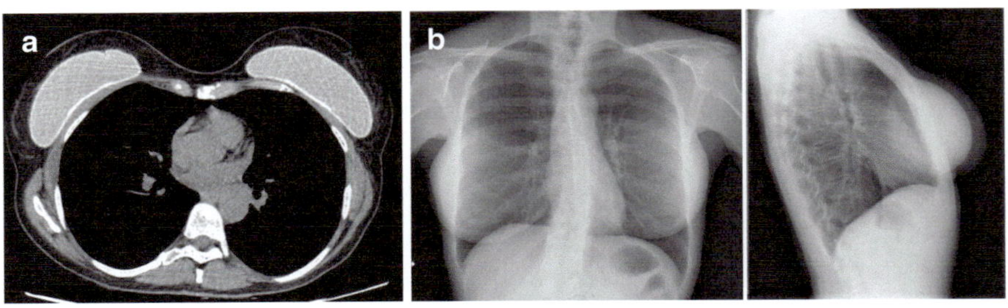

Fig. 1.2 (**a**) Chest CT scan without injection, axial slice in mediastinal window. Breast implants: the CT scan shows the presence of implants. This imaging modality does not allow a correct analysis of the implants but sometimes we incidentally discover breast masses taking the contrast, to be explored by mammography and ultrasound. (**b**) Chest X-ray front and profile. Breast implants. The patient from figure a, had the same day a chest X-ray. This technique is useless for the analysis of implants

1.1 The Elements of the Breast

The breast extends between the clavicle, the armpit, and the middle of the sternum. It is attached to the pectoralis major muscle [3].

Although also present in men, the breast is part of the female reproductive system as an accessory organ, with a larger volume of mammary gland, and especially lobules that serve to produce breast milk. In men, there is a halt in development before differentiation into the ductolobular unit, and therefore an absence of lobules.

The extension of the mammary base on the chest wall is classically described from the third intercostal space at the top, to the seventh intercostal space at the bottom. However, there is variability, and this is a theoretical description. There is no clear limit between the axillary extension of the breast, and the axilla [3].

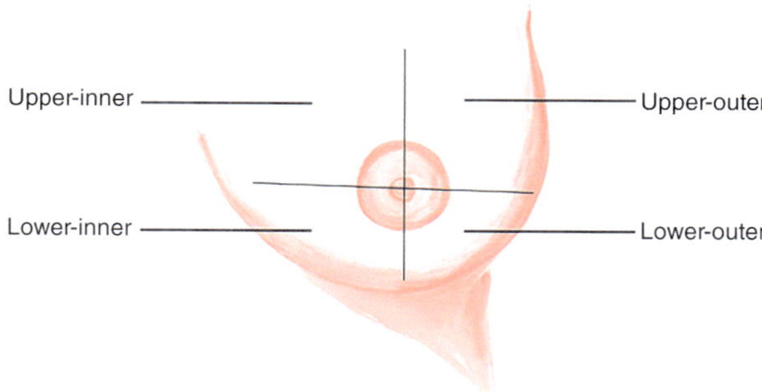

Fig. 1.3 The different quadrants of the breast: Upper-outer, Upper-inner, Lower-inner, Lower-outer. *Drawing by Jean-Charles Goldberg*

The mammary gland does not have an anterior cleavage plane with the skin, however, there is a posterior cleavage plane, constituted by the *superficialis fascia* and the aponeurosis of the pectoralis major muscle (Fig. 1.1).

The breast can be compartmentalized into four regions, each limited by a horizontal and vertical line meeting in their center at the level of the nipple (Fig. 1.3). These regions are called quadrants. The quadrants indicate the location of a pathology (upper-outer quadrant, lower-inner quadrant, union of the lower quadrants...). They do not correspond to an anatomical reality.

Different elements make up the breast:

- **The lactiferous units or lobes**: there are about fifteen. Each lobe is composed of 20 to 40 lobules and each lobule contains 10 to 100 acini.
- **The basic unit is the acinus or alveolus**. It is a rounded cavity that constitutes the secretory part of the gland and produces milk.
- **The lactiferous ducts (first and second order)**: they transport the milk from the acini to the nipple.
- **The nipple**: It is in the center of the areola, the most pigmented part of the breast. It is composed of muscle fibers that can contract and harden. It allows the milk to be evacuated.
- **The Nipple-areola complex**: It is composed of the areola and the nipple. It forms a circle, and contains sebaceous glands called areolar glands.
- **Cooper's ligaments**: they allow the fixation and support of the parenchyma to the deep part of the dermis and are composed of connective tissue.
- **Adipose tissue**: It is mixed with glandular tissue.
- **The lymphatic system**: which is detailed below.

1.2 The Lymphatic System

The breast contains a network of lymphatic vessels that allow the lymph from the breast tissues to be transported to the lymph nodes, around the mammary area.

This lymphatic system plays a role in the immune system and the healing process. Several groups of lymph nodes are involved in breast drainage [4] (Fig. 1.4):

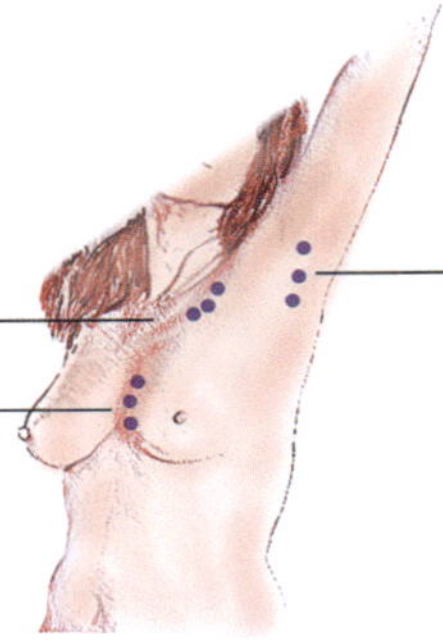

Fig. 1.4 Lymph node regions: Axillary, supraclavicular, infraclavicular, and internal mammary. *Drawing by Jean-Charles Goldberg*

1.2.1 The Axillary Lymph Nodes

They are in the axilla, with an average number from 20 to 40 in anatomical textbooks and are distributed over 3 levels depending on their position relative to the small pectoral muscle (Berg's levels) [5, 6].

- Level I: Below and external to the small pectoral muscle.
- Level II: Behind the small pectoral muscle.
- Level III: Above and medial to the small pectoral muscle.

1.2.2 The Supraclavicular Lymph Nodes

They are located above the clavicle.

1.2.3 The Subclavicular Lymph Nodes

They are located under the clavicle.

1.2.4 The Internal Mammary Lymph Nodes

They are located around the sternum, inside the thorax, near the internal mammary vessels.

References

1. Herring B, Paraskeva N, Tollow P, Harcourt D. Women's initial experiences of their appearance after mastectomy and/or breast reconstruction: a qualitative study. Psychooncology. 2019;28(10):2076–82.
2. Yalom M. A history of the breast. 1st ed. France: Galaade; 2010. p. 381.

3. Pierre Kamina. Schémas de travaux pratiques d'anatomie; planches d'anatomie Tome 24; le sein; Maloine. Aceesed 22 Dec 1998.
4. Nathalie Johnson MD, et al. Sentinel node biopsy and internal mammary lymphatic mapping in breast cancer. Am J Surg. 2000;179:386.
5. Marino MA, et al. Lymph node imaging in patients with primary breast cancer: concurrent diagnostic tools. Oncologist. 2020;25(2):e231.
6. Elisabeth W, et al. Localization of central breast lymphatics and predefined separation of lobes along the horizontal septum. Plastic Reconstruc. 2023;11:e5446.

Breast Augmentation with Implants

2

Contents

2.1 Generalities

Their use is constantly increasing [1]: 300,000 new placements per year in the United States in 2015, and about 15,000 to 30,000 per year in France currently.

S. Cohen-Zarade, *Imaging of Plastic Surgery of the Breast and Other Implants*,
https://doi.org/10.1007/978-3-031-64159-6_2

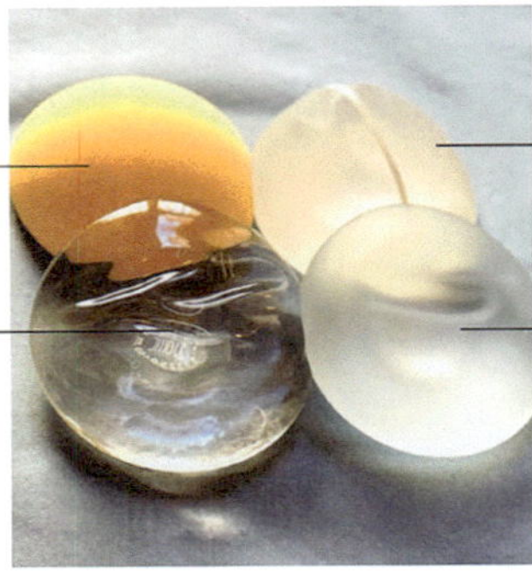

Fig. 2.1 Four different types of implants

They are placed for:

– purely aesthetic purposes in 70–80% of cases.
– in the context of a reconstruction after mastectomy in 20–30% of cases.
– for the correction of congenital malformations, such as Poland syndrome [2].

They are categorized according to the number of compartments inside, their shape, their filler material, and their envelope surface (Fig. 2.1).

2.1.1 The Compartments

Unicompartmental implant (single lumen) are the most common and almost exclusively used in recent years.

Bicompartmental implants (double lumen): the most common type is that of a central compartment inflatable filled with physiological saline, and a peripheral compartment filled with silicone (Fig. 2.2). They are often put in place during a reconstruction in patients for whom it is not possible to obtain the optimal volume immediately due to lack of skin elasticity. The saline compartment is then gradually increased by iterative injections via a subcutaneous access port to achieve the desired volume.

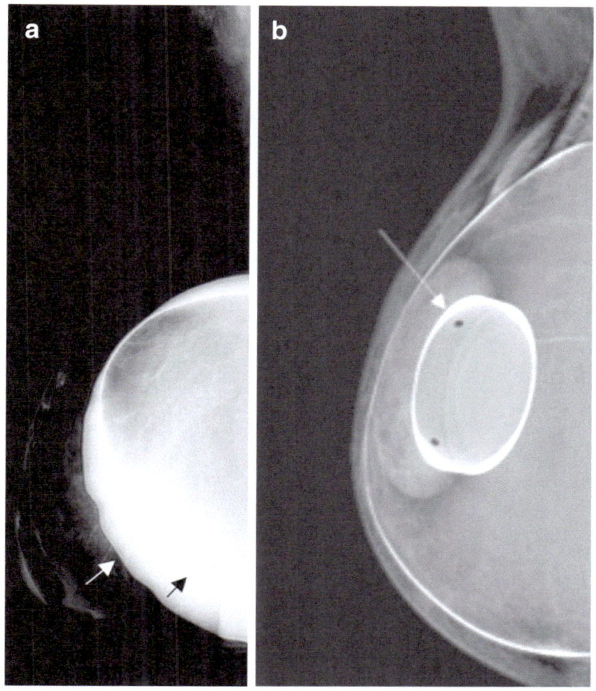

Fig. 2.2 Bicompartmental Implants. (**a**) Right mammography in oblique incidence. Bicompartmental implant. Optimized contrast for the study of the implant. It is an old implant, with two compartments, with physiological saline internally (black arrow) and silicone externally (white arrow). (**b**) Right mammography in mediolateral oblique (MLO) view (after mastectomy). Another type of an expandable implant. This implant is unicompartimental. The content is exclusively physiological saline and the valve allowing the filling of the implant (white arrow) can be seen

2.1.2 The Shape

Round implants have a symmetrical shape (Fig. 2.3).

Anatomical implants have a profiled shape, the upper part being thinner and the lower part more projected (Fig. 2.4).

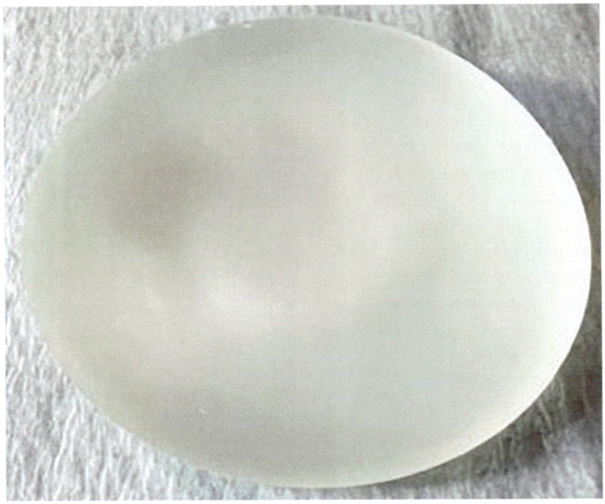

Fig. 2.3 Round implant

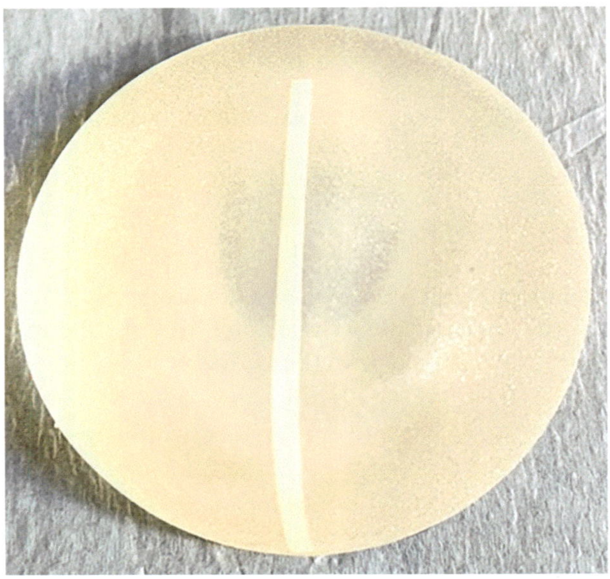

Fig. 2.4 Anatomical implant

2.1.3 The Filler Material

Implants can be pre-filled with **silicone gel** (most often), or with **physiological saline** [3].The FDA put a restriction on silicone-filled implants for cosmetic enhancement starting in 1992. However, most reconstructive patients continued to receive silicone implants post-mastectomy. This ban was put in place following concern over the risks of silicone implants. Extensive research and clinical trials did not confirm those fears of silicone. After many studies had failed to show silicone linked to diseases, the FDA, in 2006, again allowed silicone-filled implants to be used by any patient without requiring them to be enrolled in a clinical study.

2.1.4 The Envelope Surface

It is usually made of a **silicone** elastomer. It can be **smooth**, **microtextured** or **macrotextured** (Fig. 2.5). The envelope, once filled, is sealed by an occlusion tablet. The polyurethane envelope is no longer used due to the formation of a thicker capsule compared to other surface structures (Fig. 2.6).

Characteristics of an Implant

- Number of compartments: unicompartimental or bicompartimental.
- Shape: round or anatomical.
- Filler material: saline or silicone.
- Envelope surface: smooth, microtextured, or macrotextured.

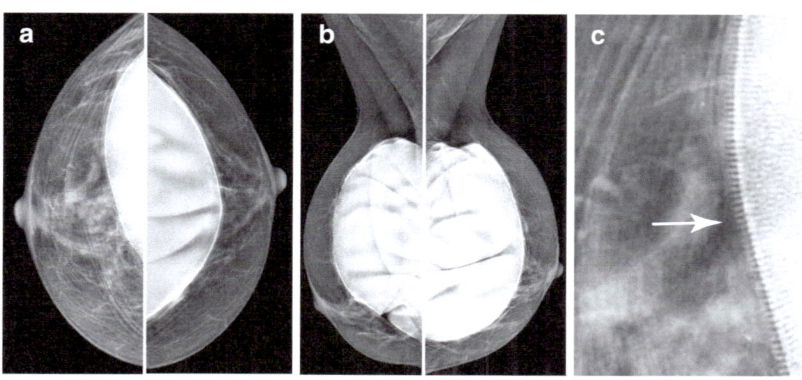

Fig. 2.5 Bilateral mammography craniocaudal (CC) view (**a**), MLO (**b**) and zoomed view (**c**). Round macro-textured implant in retroglandular position. The envelope is clearly visible "bristling" (white arrow on the zoomed view)

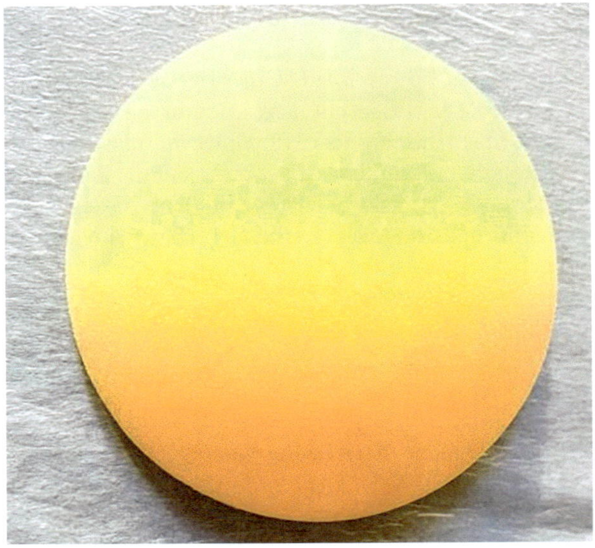

Fig. 2.6 Implant with polyurethane envelope

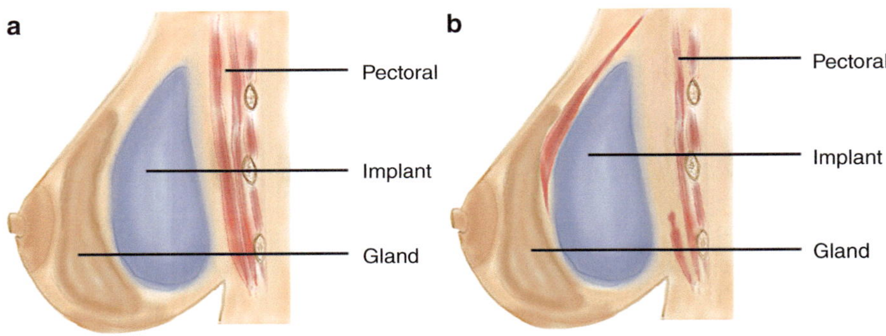

Fig. 2.7 Anatomical view of a breast in profile with different positions of an implant. (**a**) The implant is under the gland and pre-pectoral. (**b**) The implant is under-pectoral. *Drawings by Jean-Charles Goldberg*

The positioning is described in relation to the pectoralis major muscle (Fig. 2.7):

- **pre-pectoral**: the implant is retro-glandular (Fig. 2.7a),
- **retro-pectoral**: the implant is retro-pectoral (Fig. 2.7b),
- **in Dual Plane**: the upper part of the implant is under the pectoral; the lower part is under the gland.

The placement of the implant induces a normal local inflammatory reaction, resulting in the immediate formation of a fibrous peri-prosthetic capsule 1–1.5 mm thick.

It should be noted that the clinical examination is essential and rather contributory in the presence of implants: the implant increases the sensitivity of the clinical examination. Indeed, the mammary gland being always in front of the implant, it is "compacted" between the implant and the skin, and a mass is easily perceptible.

2.2 Imaging Assessment

2.2.1 Imaging Protocol

The Standard Pre-Surgical Assessment

It includes a mammography with two 2D views (CC and MLO), a tomosynthesis acquisition, and an ultrasound if needed.

Any lesion classified as ACR4, ACR5 or even ACR3 must be biopsied for histological analysis before surgery [4].

There is no consensus, but most surgeons prefer a normal mammography from 6 months to 1 year old before the intervention.

The age of realization is mandatory after 40 years and debatable before, but we almost always take a single MLO view of each breast between 30 and 40 years, in addition to the ultrasound, in search of microcalcifications [4].

The Follow-up

It is identical to that of the general population. The risk of developing breast cancer is the same in patients with implants as in others [2].

It is also recommended to perform an annual ultrasound surveillance of implants placed more than 5 years ago, or even before, in case of a change in their appearance.

The MRI

It has a sensitivity of 72–94% and a specificity of 85–97% for the detection of breast implant ruptures [5]. It is more sensitive and more specific than mammography and ultrasound but reserved for symptomatic patients or with a standard assessment suggesting a rupture. It is not recommended to perform an MRI in the systematic follow-up of patients with implants.

Imaging Protocol

- Preoperative assessment dating from 6 months to 1 year prior to the procedure.
- Follow-up identical to that of the general population or annual ultrasound 5 years post-implantation if the patient is under 40 years of age.
- MRI not routinely required preoperatively or for follow-up.

2.2.2 Mammography

The effectiveness of mammography in women with breast implants is reduced, but adjusting acquisition parameters, using advanced reconstruction algorithms, performing additional mammographic views (Fig. 2.8), and utilizing ultrasound can compensate for this decrease in efficacy.

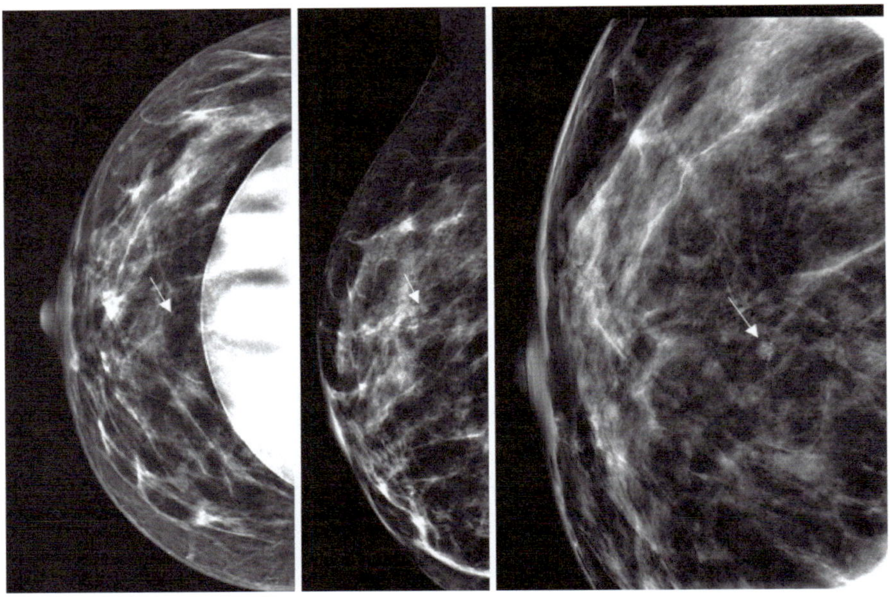

Fig. 2.8 Right mammography CC view, LM and zoomed view on the initial CC view: We visualize, with the implant displaced, a faint small round focus of microcalcifications of 2 mm, at the union of the upper quadrants. The additional profile and magnification views performed in the same way as for a patient without an implant, show better the numerous and discreetly polymorphic microcalcifications. The patient benefited from a DBT guided biopsy, which showed a low-grade ductal carcinoma in situ (DCIS)

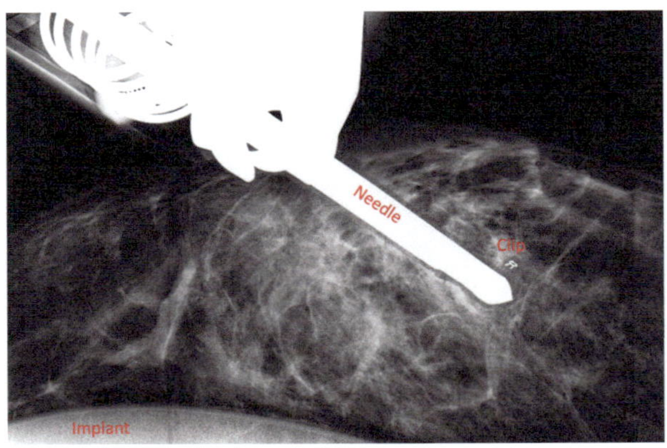

Fig. 2.9 Mammography after DBT guided biopsy for control of the accurate clip placement: The implant has been pushed back, away from the cluster of microcalcifications. At each step of the procedure, the control views prevent damage to the implant

Additional mammographic views such as the lateromedial view (LM) or the magnification views, are performed in the same way as without implants (Fig. 2.8).

Similarly, stereotactic macrobiopsy or digital breast tomosynthesis (DBT) guided biopsy, can be performed in the same way as without implants, by pushing the implant as far as possible out of the sampling window (Fig. 2.9).

Incidences: craniocaudal view (CC), lateromedial oblique view (LMO) and tomosynthesis.

One of the 2D incidences must be performed with the Eklund technique. Generally, we choose the CC view.

Tomosynthesis is often performed in LM view, to have an additional view.

The Eklund Technique (Fig. 2.10).

The implant is pushed back, and the mammary gland is pulled forward, under the compression paddle, for a better analysis of the parenchyma. The goal is to compress as much gland as possible. At most, the implant is not even visible on the view.

It is estimated that in the case of a retroglandular implant, the risk of masked tissue is 45%, versus 36% with the Eklund technique. In the case of a retropectoral implant, the risk of masked tissue is 25%, versus 15% with the Eklund technique [6].

If the technique is correctly performed, the delivered dose is the same as in the absence of an implant.

The oblique incidence is performed at high kilovoltage, with less compression, for analysis of the implant.

However, adjusting the acquisition parameters specifically for implants and utilizing specialized reconstruction algorithms helps to minimize the delivered dose, achieving a level almost equivalent to that of mammography without an implant.

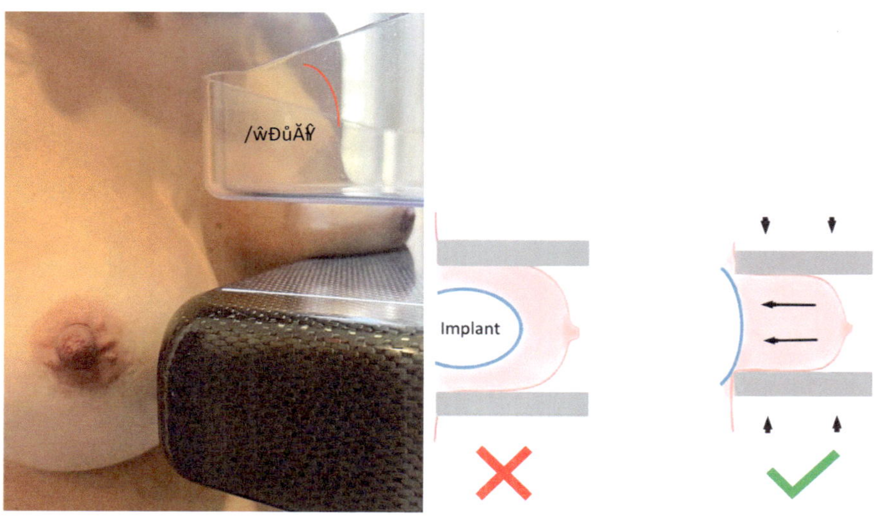

Fig. 2.10 Photo and diagram of the Eklund technique, pushing the implant back from the mammography compression paddle

On the console, thanks to the digital system, by modifying the windowing, the contrast can be optimized differently. We can choose to analyze the mammary parenchyma or the implant (Fig. 2.11).

It is thus possible to reveal through a silicone implant, details previously invisible on a traditional film.

> Note that we have never observed a rupture of the implant after performing a mammography.

Tomosynthesis is more difficult to interpret than without an implant, because the mammary parenchyma is compacted between the skin and the implant, but it remains complementary to standard views.

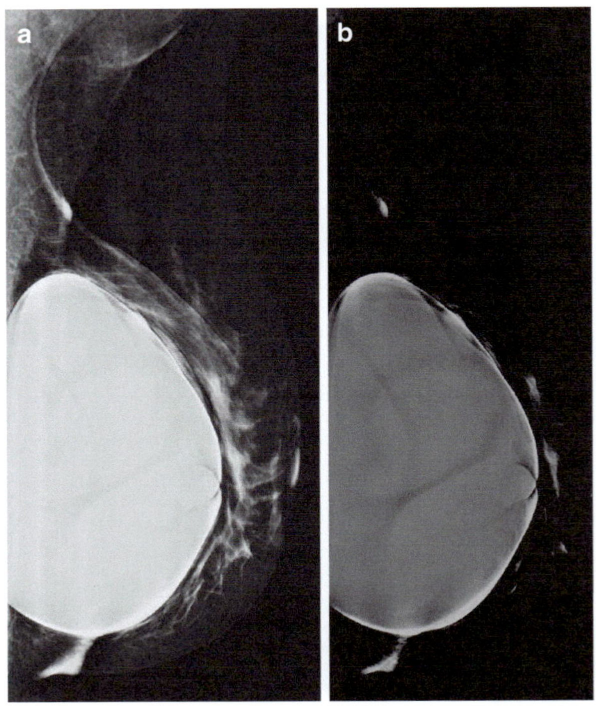

Fig. 2.11 Mammography of the left breast in LMO view. Two different visualization settings on the reading console, showing more optimally the mammary parenchyma (**a**) and the implant with its black folds (**b**)

Standards Views

- CC view with Eklund technique.
- LMO view.
- Tomosynthesis.

The basic analysis is:

- Appearance of the implant: it is oval, with regular edges and a homogeneous content.
- Its position: retropectoral (Figs. 2.12 and 2.13) or prepectoral and retroglandular (Figs. 2.5, 2.14 and 2.15). It is clearly distinguished on the MLO view.

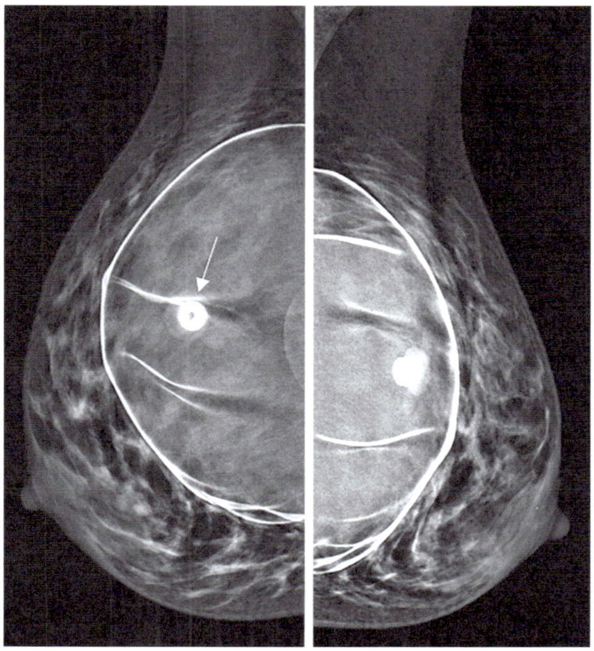

Fig. 2.12 Bilateral mammography in MLO view: Retromuscular round saline-filled implants. The occlusion tablet is clearly visible

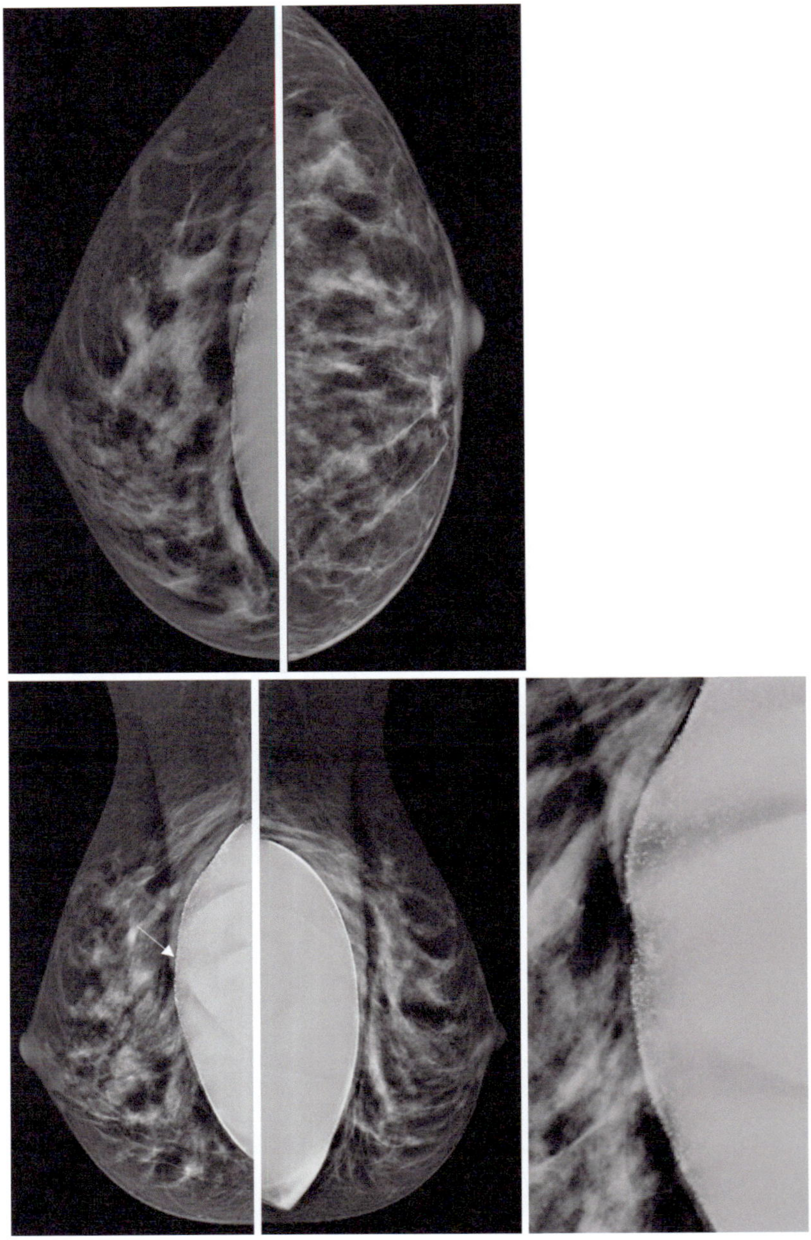

Fig. 2.13 Bilateral mammography, 2 views and zoomed views. Calcifications of the envelope surface. Anatomical silicone-filled implants in a retropectoral position. Non-pathological calcifications of the implant wall on the right are noticed, which can appear over time. It is also noticed that the Eklund technique was more easily achievable on the left, where the implant is completely pushed back so that it is no longer visible on the CC view

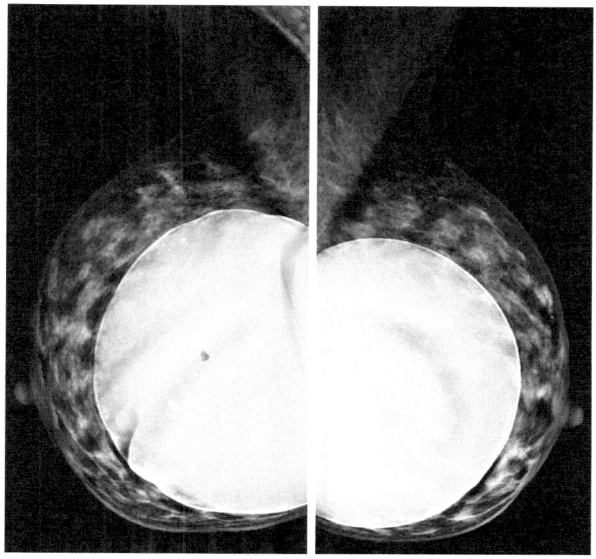

Fig. 2.14 Bilateral mammography in MLO view. PIP implants. Round silicone-filled implants in a retroglandular position of the PIP type (suspended from the market due to a higher number of ruptures than other manufacturers)

We also sometimes visualize the markers of anatomical implants, witnesses of the centering in the breast, ideally located at the junction between the external and internal quadrants (Fig. 2.16 and 2.17).

- Its shape: round (Figs. 2.5, 2.12 and 2.14) or anatomical (Figs. 2.13, 2.15 and 2.18).
- Its content:

Silicone appears dense, very opaque with black folds visualized within the implant by changing the contrast on the reading console (Figs. 2.5, 2.13, 2.14 and 2.15).

Physiological saline is less dense (Fig. 2.12). The mammary parenchyma and the posterior aspect of the implant (occlusion tablet) are visible through transparency.

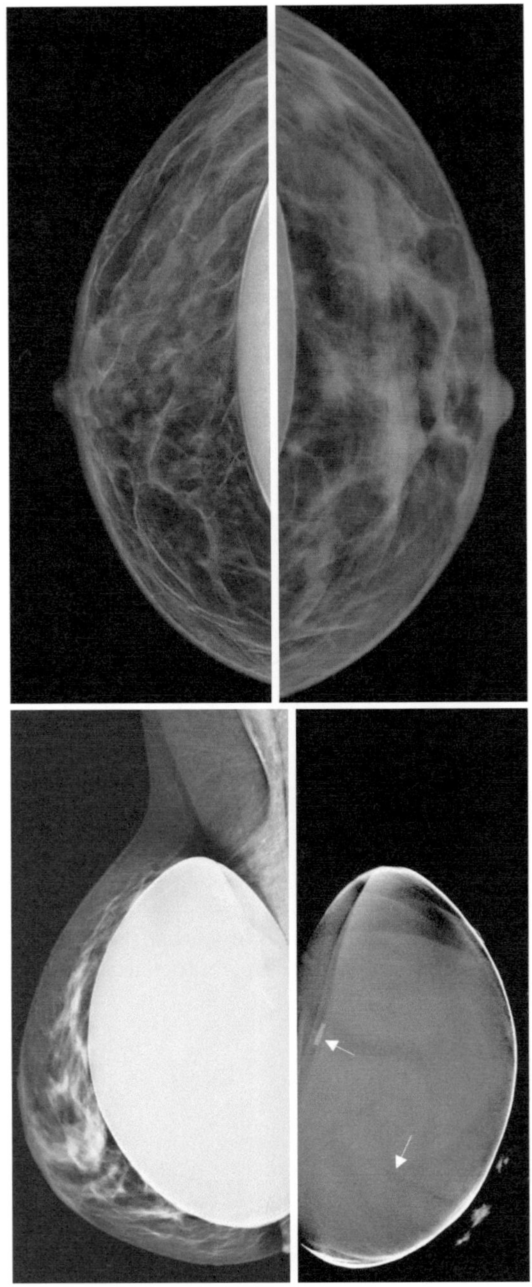

Fig. 2.15 Bilateral mammography with two views. Intact anatomical implants in a retroglandular position. On the CC view, with Eklund technique, the gland was pulled forward as much as possible. Note that the contrast on the left oblique shot of this image is optimized for the implant study. The folds and the posterior occlusion tablet (arrows) can be distinguished

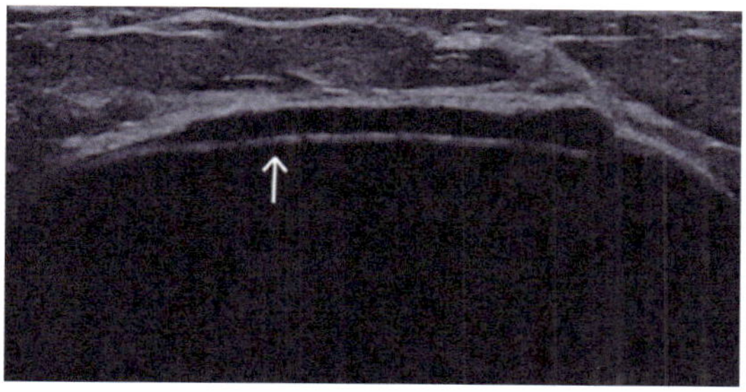
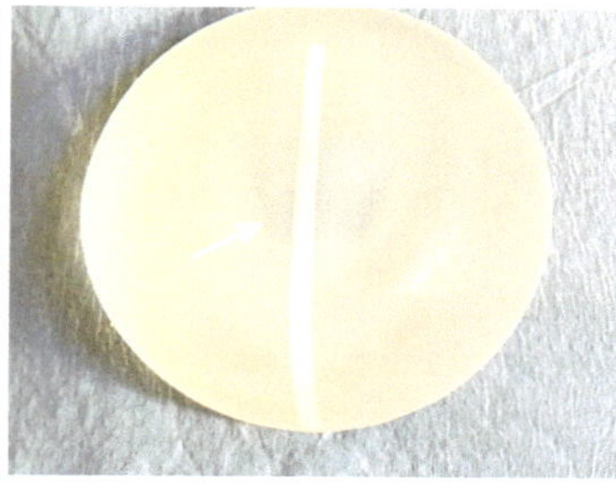

Fig. 2.16 Breast ultrasound longitudinal section and photo of an anatomical implant: Anatomical marker. Trap: Normal "Tab" serving as an anatomical marker, for the positioning of the implant. The capsulo-membranous complex remains intact. The contralateral aspect is the same

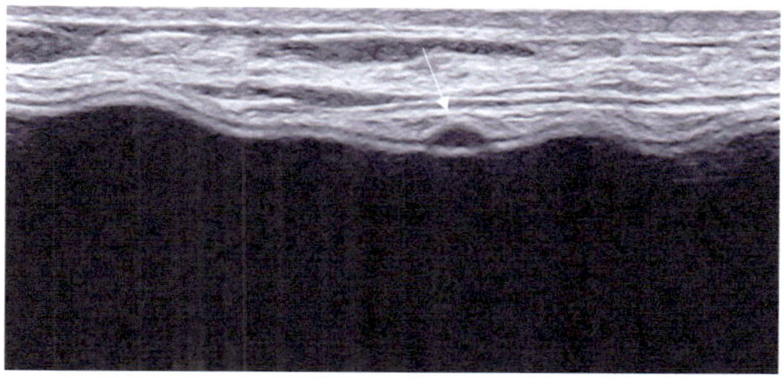

Fig. 2.17 Breast ultrasound: Normal anatomical marker. It presents as a small bulge. Up to three successive ones can be seen aligned

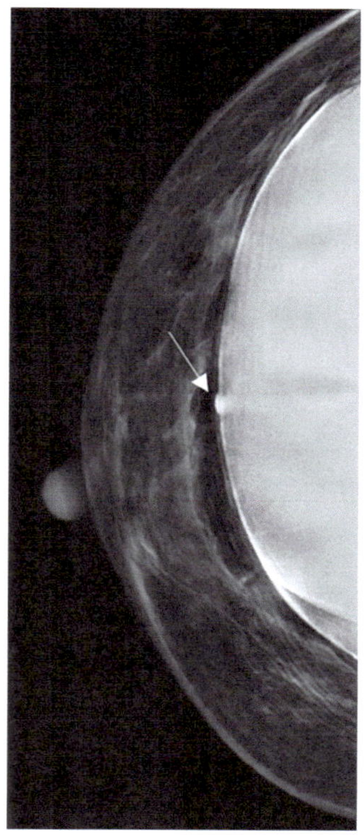

Fig. 2.18 Right mammography. CC view. Anatomical marker. Intact and well-placed anatomical silicone-filled implant. An anatomical marker perfectly centered can be seen

2.2.3 Ultrasound

It is systematically performed in the presence of implants, even in the case of breasts of low density, type a or b, as defined by the Birads classification.

Execution

The examination is operator dependent.

Like any ultrasound procedure, it involves a learning curve. The analysis should be conducted in two stages: initially, examining the gland to search for lesions (Fig. 2.19), and subsequently, inspecting the implant with different settings. This includes adjusting the depth of the focal point to look for any complications associated with the implant.

These two distinct examination times are necessary in order not to overlook an anomaly.

Care must be taken with the reverberation artifact of the anterior surface of the implant and these echoes must be removed without masking any real signs of rupture (Fig. 2.20).

It is also necessary to compare the right and left sides (Fig. 2.17).

Analysis

A good homogeneous adjustment shows:

- A well-defined capsule-envelope complex, represented by hyperechoic lines, two or three in number depending on the implants, parallel and adjoining (Figs. 2.21, 2.22, 2.23, 2.24, 2.25 and 2.26).
- A homogeneous content of the implant, purely anechoic, either because it is liquid (Fig. 2.21), or because it is silicone. In both cases, it is transversed by ultrasound waves". (Figs. 2.22, 2.23 and 2.24).
- Harmoniously arranged physiological radial folds are observed (Fig. 2.25). It is common to find a thin layer of fluid surrounding the implant, which often extends into these folds.

A classic trap is the bulge formed by the "anatomical markers "or "tabs "of anatomical implants (useful for perioperative centering), which is a normal aspect and should not raise suspicion of a beginning of rupture, with separation of the hyperechoic lines. The identical contralateral aspect reinforces the diagnostic certainty (Fig. 2.16).

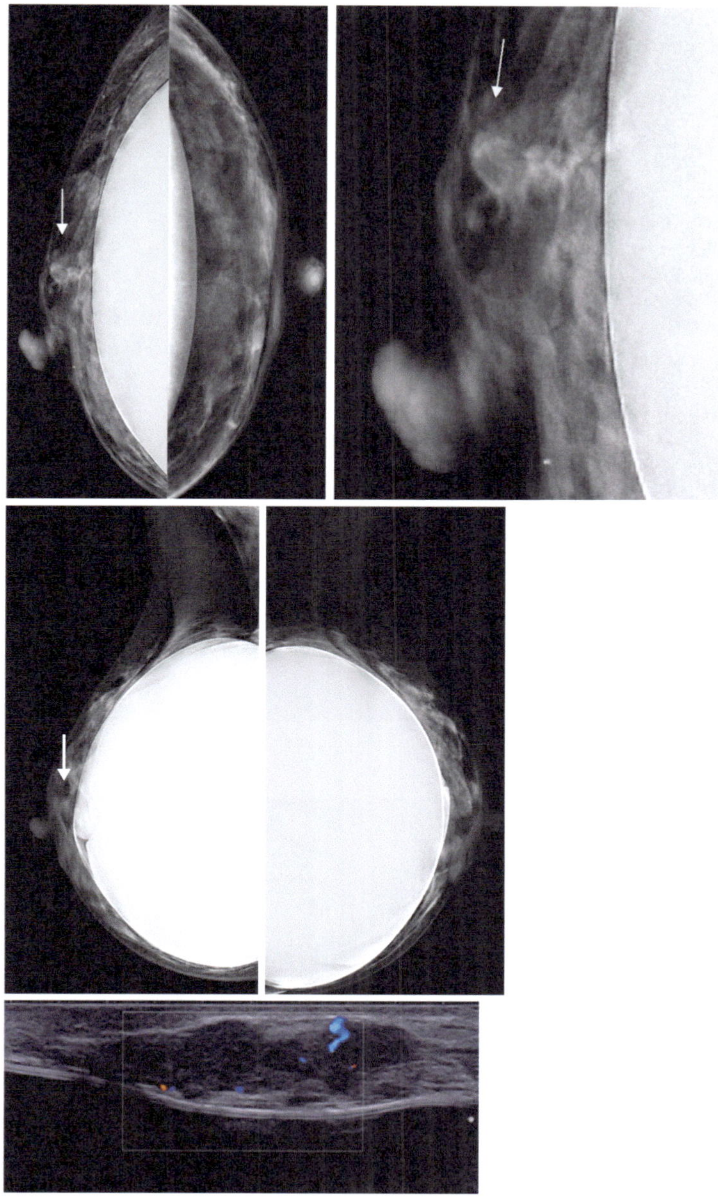

Fig. 2.19 Bilateral mammography and right breast ultrasound with color doppler. Infiltrating ductal carcinoma. On the mammography, especially on the right CC view, there is a poorly defined mass in the upper-outer quadrant (arrow). Additional views, such as spot views, are difficult to perform due to the large volume of the implants and the thin glandular thickness. The ultrasound finds the hypoechoic mass, poorly defined, with indistincts contours, hypervascularized, in the upper-outer quadrant, more evident than on the mammography. Note that the silicone-filled retromuscular implants are intact

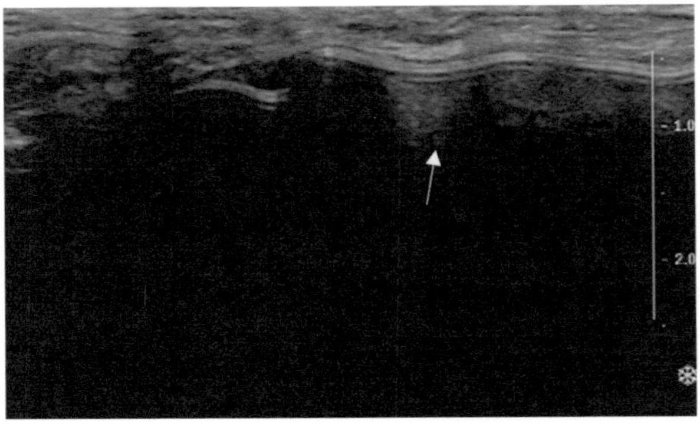

Fig. 2.20 Breast ultrasound. Incorrect ultrasound settings. Silicone-filled implant intact. Incorrect ultrasound settings, causing the appearance of reverberation artifacts of the anterior surface of the implant. However, the capsulo-membranous complex is perfectly continuous

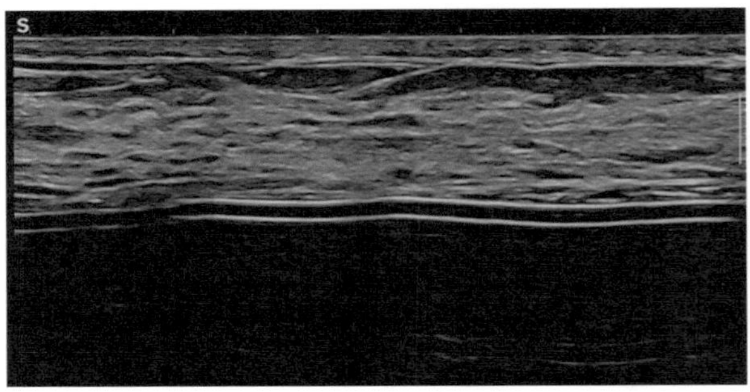

Fig. 2.21 Breast ultrasound. Intact saline-filled implant. Capsulo-membranous complex forming two non-adjoining but perfectly parallel hyperechoic lines. The content appears anechoic, liquid

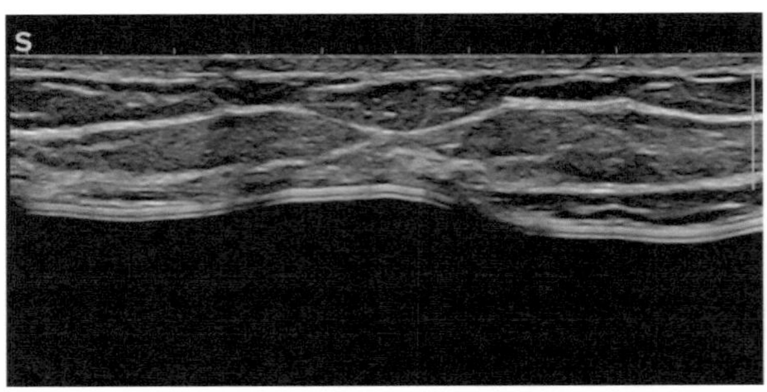

Fig. 2.22 Breast ultrasound. Intact silicone-filled implant. The normal capsulo-membranous complex is visible, in the form of 3 adjoining hyperechoic lines. The content appears anechoic, homogeneous

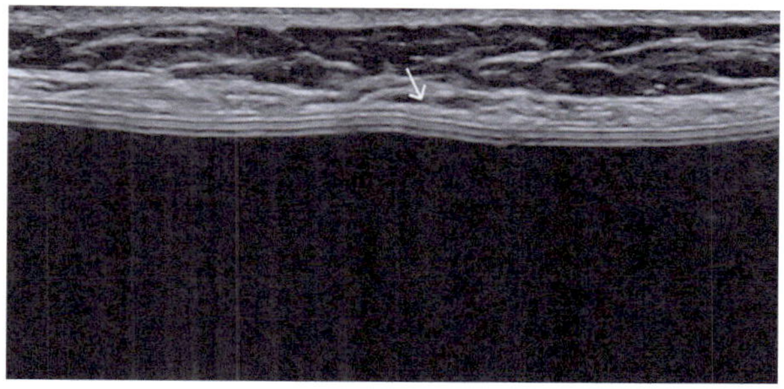

Fig. 2.23 Breast ultrasound. Normal capsulo-membranous complex in the form of 3 adjoining hyperechoic lines. This is a different implant brand than the previous image (Fig. 2.22) and the layers do not have the same appearance

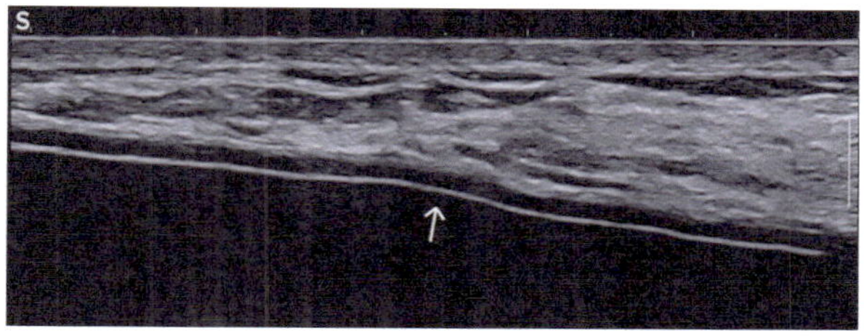

Fig. 2.24 Breast ultrasound. Intact PIP implant. The capsulo-membranous complex is represented by two hyperechoic lines quite like that of a saline implant

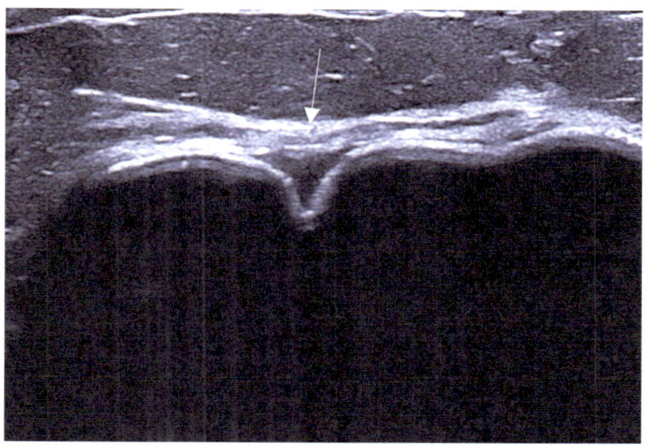

Fig. 2.25 Breast ultrasound. Radial fold. Normal implant fold with physiological liquid effusion at this level

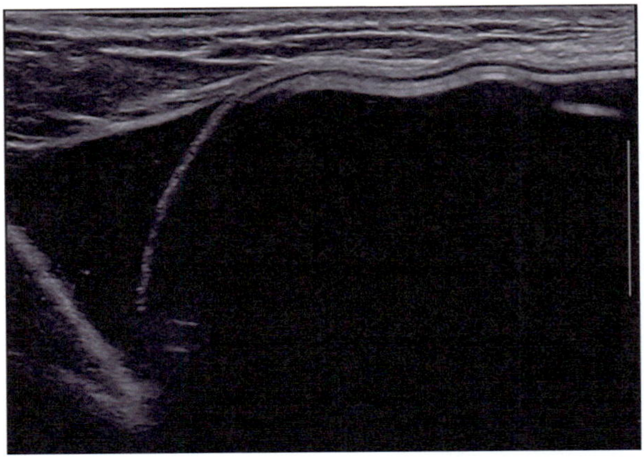

Fig. 2.26 Breast ultrasound. Intact bicompartimental implant. Content of physiological saline and silicone. Several parallel folds between them, corresponding to the envelopes of the internal and external compartments. The intact continuity of the capsulo-membranous complex, along with a comparison to the patient's previous examinations, allows us to confirm the absence of rupture

Normal Appearance of an Implant on Ultrasound

- Adherence of the hyperechoic lines of the capsulo-membranous complex.
- Homogeneous anechoic content.
- Some physiological radial folds.

The ultrasound-guided microbiopsy can be performed in the same way as without implants, sometimes with the help of the injected anesthetic to move the lesion away from the implant.

2.2.4 MRI

This is the reference examination to evaluate the integrity of silicone breast implants. Its sensitivity for rupture detection is 72–94% and its specificity is 85 to 97% [6].

A dedicated breast antenna is used, with the patient in the prone position, the breasts placed in the space of each antenna. It is performed in the second week of the menstrual cycle to minimize background glandular enhancement.

Acquisition Protocol

- **Axial T2-weighted sequence** with or without Fat sat (FSE/TSE) or Axial T2 DIXON (4 T2-weighted sequences with and without fat signal saturation). The slice thickness is 3.6 mm, and the sequence lasts about 3 min.
- **Dedicated "Silicone only" sequence** if the implant is silicone-filled: on this sequence, only the silicone is in high signal, everything else is black: It is a STIR-weighted sequence with fat signal suppression and a spectral suppression of the water signal.
- **Dynamic T1-weighted sequence before and after intravenous administration of a gadolinium chelate** (0.1 mmol/kg at a rate of 2–3 mL/s) and with subtraction for better contrast uptake analysis: 3D EG T1 with or without fat signal saturation. The slice thickness is 0.7 mm. The first sequence after injection is performed between 1.5 and 2 min and the last at about 6 min.
- The diffusion-weighted sequence (DWI) is reserved for cancer indications.
- The duration of the examination is 15–20 min. There are currently ultra-fast protocols that allow to reduce it.

> If the "silicone only" sequence is not contributive and the patient is unsure about the content of the implant, it is very likely a saline prosthesis.

Except in the case of a very young patient, even if the prescriber's request is to look for a prosthetic complication, we must not forget the analysis of the breast parenchyma and the search for a tumor.

In practice, we perform an injection from the age of 35, or even before, if there is a family risk factor or a genetic mutation.

The latest version of the *Atlas Breast Imaging-Reporting and Data System* (BI-RADS) from the *American College of Radiology* (ACR) was published in the United States at the end of 2013 and includes implants and their characteristics in MRI (Table 2.1).

Analysis

- **Implant contours**: The membrane appears continuous, completely adhered to the fibrous peri-prosthetic capsule, in the form of a hypointense line. There are some radial folds: They are common, regardless of the type of implant, and extend from the periphery to the center of the implant (Fig. 2.27), in the form of a thick hypointense line.

They are generally simple and few but sometimes longer and multidirectional. They are the main cause of diagnostic error in intracapsular rupture. There may also be small bulges or small focal hernias.

Table 2.1 Birads MRI of implants. Extracted from ACR BI-RADS® Atlas Fifth Edition of the American College of Radiology

Implants
(a) **Implant material and lumen type**
Saline
Silicone
Intact ruptured
Other implant material (such as soy oil, polypropylene; polyurethane and sponges: Includes direct injections)
Lumen type
(b) **Implant location**
Retroglandular
Retropectoral
(c) **Abnormal implant contour**
Focal bulge
(d) **Intracapsular silicone findings**
Radial folds
Subcapsular line
Keyhole sign (teardrop, noose)
Linguine sign
(e) **Extracapsular silicone**
Breast
Lymph node
(f) **Water droplets**
(g) **Peri implant fluid**

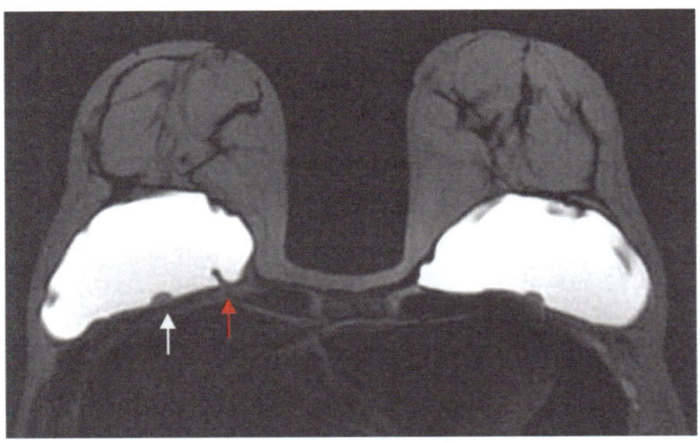

Fig. 2.27 Breast MRI. Radial folds. "Silicone-only" sequence. The silicone-filled implants in retropectoral position appear intact. The posterior occlusion disc (white arrow) and some normal folds (red arrow) are observed

- **Its content**: of saline or silicone. It should be homogeneous.

  Silicone appears as intermediate (gray) signal on T1 and T2, and as high signal on the 'silicone only' sequence, without contrast enhancement (Fig. 2.28). Saline appears as low signal on T1, clear high signal on T2, low signal on the 'silicone only' sequence, without contrast enhancement (Fig. 2.29).

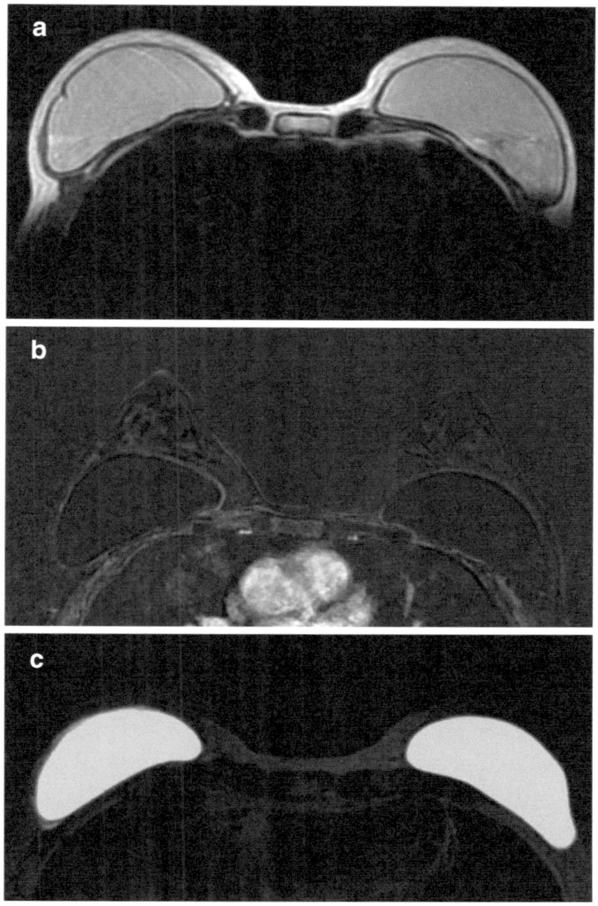

Fig. 2.28 Breast MRI. Retroglandular silicone-filled implant. (**a**): T2-weighted sequence, (**b**): T1-weighted FS sequence after injection, at 2 min, (**c**): WATER STIR "silicone only" sequence. The implants are intact. The silicone appears as a clear hyperintensity on the "silicone only" sequence

- **Its position**: retroglandular (Fig. 2.28) or retropectoral (Fig. 2.27). The pectoral muscle is clearly visible and followed along its entire path and the position of the implant is easily identifiable.
- **The presence of a peri-prosthetic effusion**: It is common and physiological if it is of low abundance. It is often found in relation to a fold. It appears as a T2 hyperintense signal.

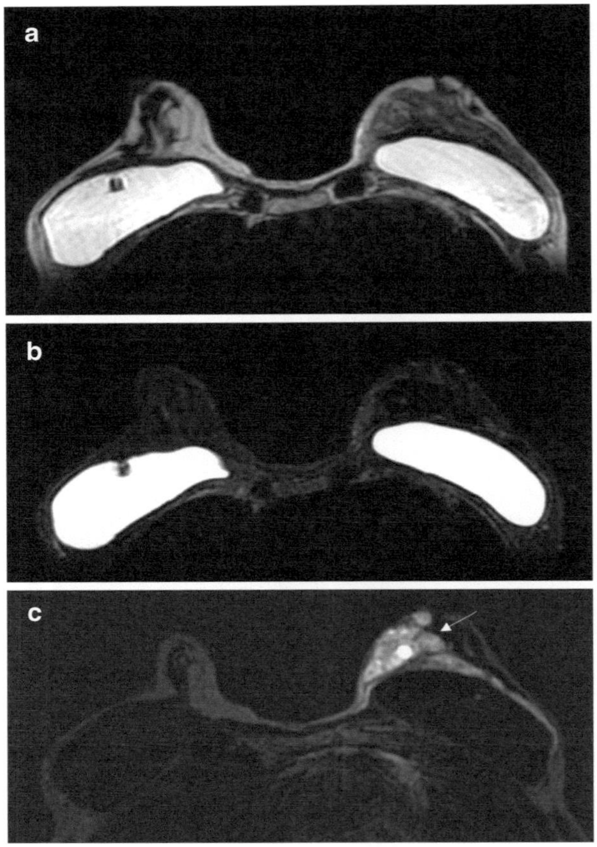

Fig. 2.29 Breast MRI. T2-weighted sequence (**a**), T2-weighted fat-suppressed (**b**), and “silicone only” (**c**). Saline implants and residual siliconomas. The intact saline implants, in retropectoral position, appear as T2 hyperintensity and hypointensity on the sequence dedicated to silicone. Note that on this last sequence, the confluent hyperintense masses of the left breast correspond to siliconomas from a previous explanted implant (arrow). Except in this special case, the “silicone only” sequence is not necessary for women who have never had a silicone implant

2.3 Complications of Breast Implants

The different complications are rupture (intra or extra-capsular), capsular contracture, effusion, rotation, siliconic lymph node, and anaplastic large cell lymphoma (BIA-ALCL).

2.3.1 Rupture

This is the most common complication in imaging, as it is the first cause of implant removal [7]. Its risk of occurrence increases with the age of the implant, with an average delay of 7.6 years [1].

The rupture rate is 15% at 10 years for third generation of implants [8].

There are two types of ruptures in relation to the fibrous peri-prosthetic capsule:

The intracapsular rupture (ICR), representing between 80 and 90% of ruptures and the extracapsular rupture (ECR) between 10 and 20%.

The evolution is possible from an ICR to an ECR, but not systematic, in 1–3 years [1].

Historically, it was believed that implants needed to be replaced every 10 years. However, this approach is now subject to debate. In the absence of complications, without any FDA (Food and Drug Administration) recommendations for the removal of a specific type of implant, and if the aesthetic result remains satisfactory, there is no need to replace the implants.

Intracapsular Rupture (ICR)

It is rarely related to trauma but rather due to a spontaneous weakening of the envelope [9]. It concerns all silicone-filled gel implants and represents most ruptures. It involves a silicone leak through the prosthetic membrane to the fibrous capsule, formed by the body during the implant placement. There is no silicone in the rest of the breast. Gradually, the prosthetic envelope collapses and floats within the silicone gel. It may be associated with homolateral axillary or internal mammary siliconic lymph nodes. It is almost always asymptomatic. It is in no way painful and there is no loss of breast volume. It slowly evolves towards extracapsular rupture and requires a non-urgent prosthetic change (within the year).

In imaging:

Mammography

It can show (Figs. 2.30 and 2.31):

- An implant with deformed contours as it spreads within its capsule. It appears enlarged, sometimes exhibiting a pseudo double contour, and loses its ovoid shape with defined edges.
- White folds, in contrast with the normal black folds.
- A heterogeneous content, with typically small bubbles called “salad oil“, within the dense silicone.

The view, in MLO, optimized for the study of the implant, with a higher kilovoltage, is the most suitable for visualizing these three signs. The contrast must be adjusted during the analysis on the console to highlight the folds. Tomosynthesis does not contribute to the diagnosis [8].

ICR on Mammography

- Deformed contours.
- White folds.
- Heterogeneous content.

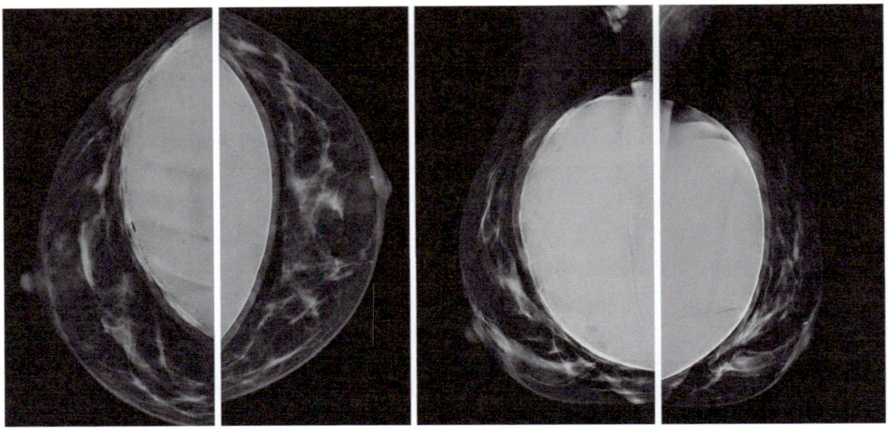

Fig. 2.30 Bilateral mammography CC and MLO. ICR. On the right, there is an irregularity of the implant contours, a heterogeneous content and white folds related to an intracapsular rupture. Note the homolateral siliconic axillary lymph nodes

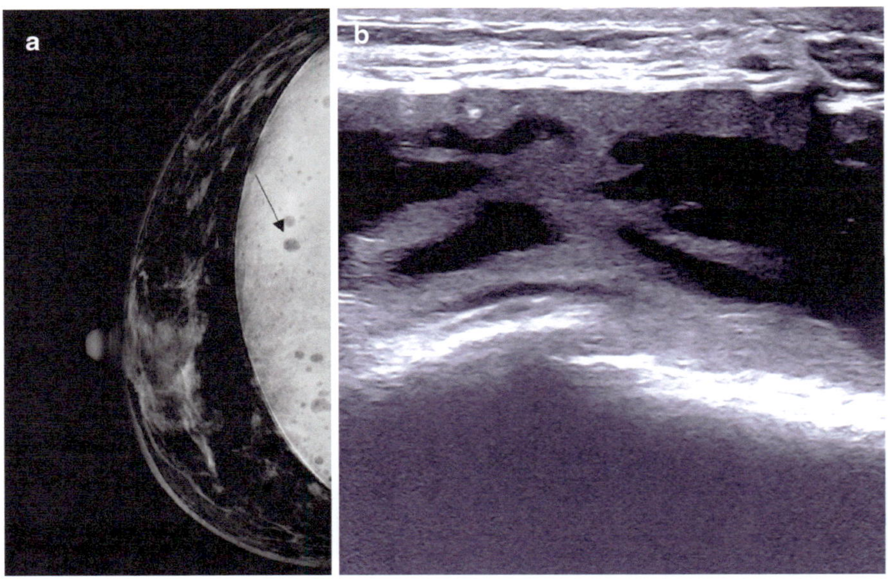

Fig. 2.31 Mammography and ultrasound of the right breast. Advanced ICR. Highly heterogeneous content of the right implant on mammography (**a**) and on the ultrasound image (**b**), with the presence of liquid bubbles (black arrow)

Ultrasound [10]: There is typically a spacing or detachment of the hyperechoic lines between the prosthetic membrane and the capsule, with silicone insinuated between the two. This aspect is easily distinguished from reverberation echoes by optimizing the settings. An early and strictly posterior intracapsular rupture may be overlooked because ultrasound does not properly penetrate the silicone and the posterior membrane is not visible (Figs. 2.32 and 2.33).

We can also see a heterogeneous content of the prosthesis, which loses its completely homogeneous anechoic appearance (Fig. 2.31).

ICR on Ultrasound

- Detachment of the hyperechoic lines of the capsulo-membranous complex.
- Heterogeneous content.

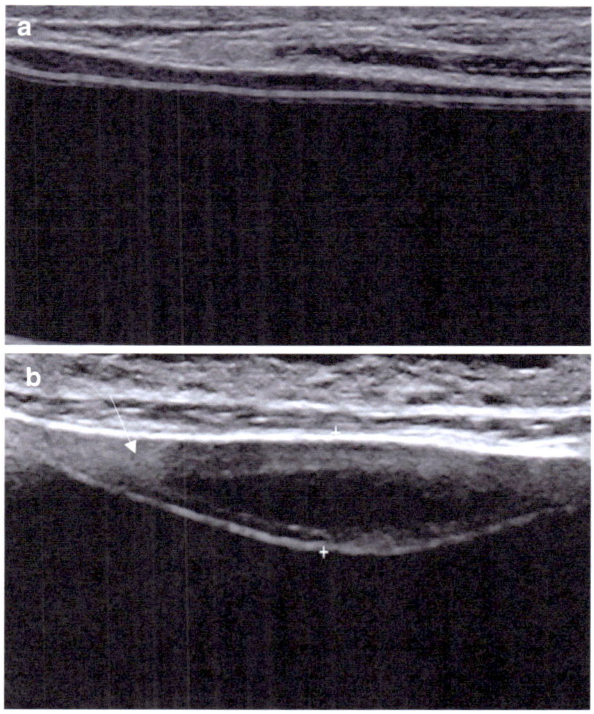

Fig. 2.32 Right (**a**) and left (**b**) breast ultrasound. ICR. Normal appearance on the right. On the left, detachment of the hyperechoic lines between the prosthetic membrane and the capsule, with a fluid containing silicone insinuated between the two

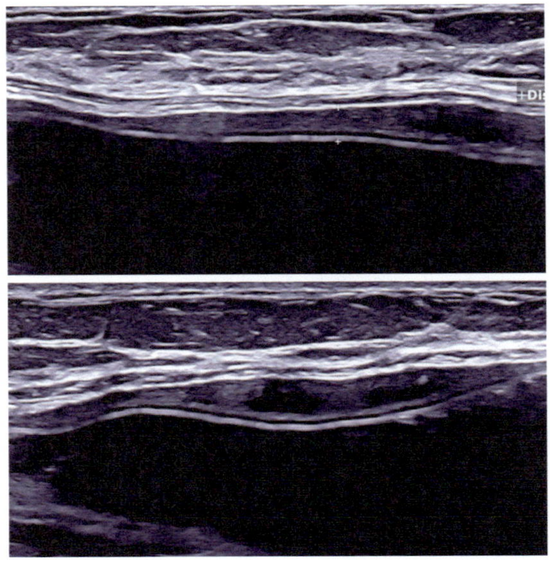

Fig. 2.33 Left breast ultrasound.
ICR. Detachment of the hyperechoic lines between the prosthetic membrane and the capsule, with an effusion containing silicone insinuated between the two

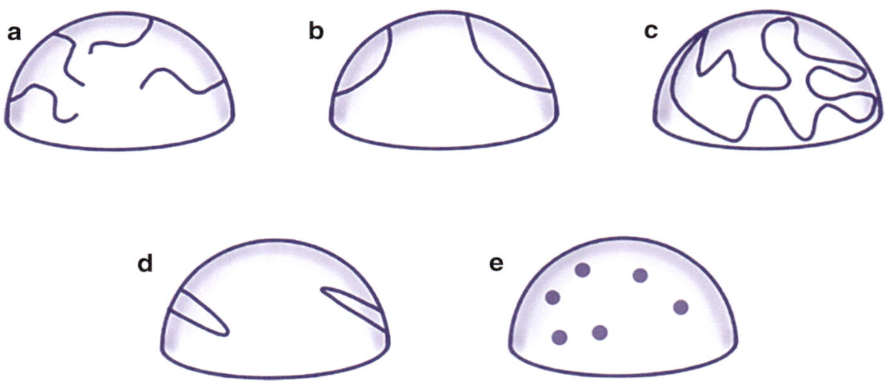

Fig. 2.34 Diagrams of silicone-filled gel implants in MRI. (**a**) Normal folds; (**b**) Beginning ICR; (**c**) "Linguine sign"; (**d**) "Keyhole" appearance; (**e**) "Salad oil"appearance with heterogeneous content

MRI

This is the most sensitive examination for diagnosis.

The WATER-STIR-weighted sequence dedicated to silicone must be performed, in addition to standard sequences of the breast MRI protocol [6].

We describe:

- The "linguine sign": This is the most typical appearance. It looks like a spaghetti or like strands of linguine pasta, corresponding to stacked membranous layers, in hyposignal, within the implant in hypersignal on the WATER-STIR -weighted sequence (Fig. 2.34: diagrams b becoming c, Figs. 2.35 and 2.36).

  They should not be confused with the normal folds that connect to the wall (Fig. 2.34: diagram a, Fig. 2.37).

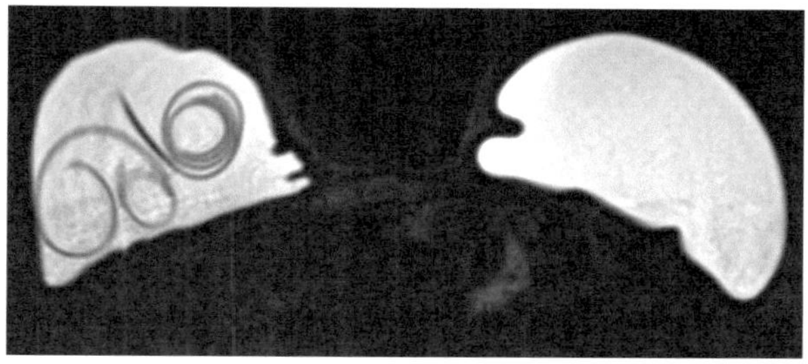

Fig. 2.35 Breast MRI "silicone only" sequence. ICR. On the right, there is a characteristic linguine sign. There is no extracapsular silicone. The left implant is intact

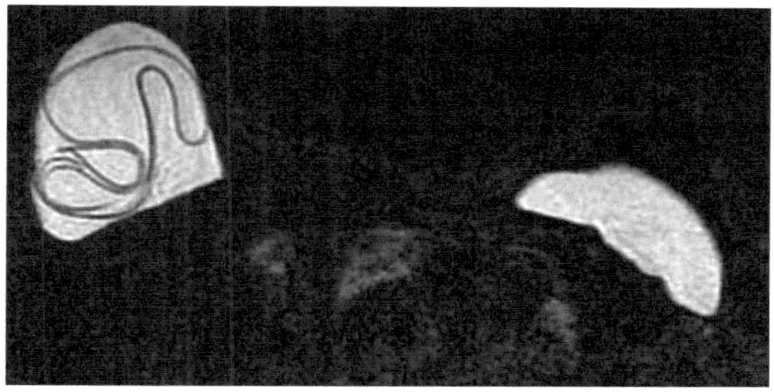

Fig. 2.36 Breast MRI "silicone only" sequence. ICR. On the right: characteristic linguine sign. There is no extracapsular silicone. The left implant is intact

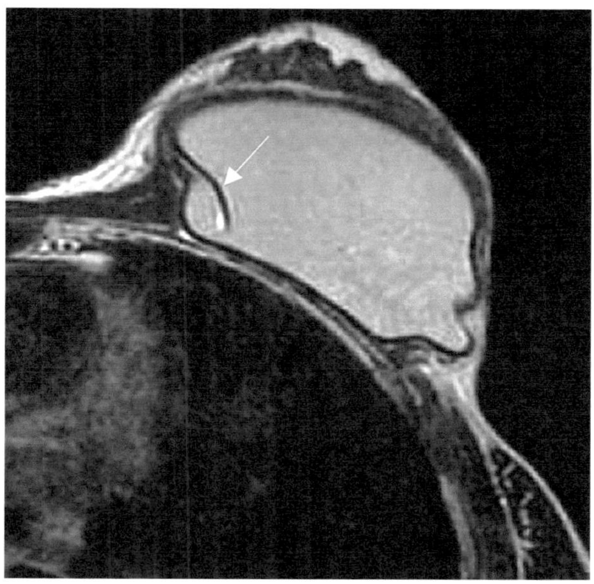

Fig. 2.37 Breast MRI focused on the left breast, T2-weighted sequence. Normal implant fold (arrow). We see the membranous connection

- At a minimum, we can see a "perspiration"of silicone through the membrane, without it floating, comparable to the splitting of the two hyperechoic lines of the capsulo-membranous complex in ultrasound (Fig. 2.38).
- The "keyhole"appearance, or "noose"or even "teardrop": This is a small splitting of the prosthetic membrane with silicone inserted at this level, between the two membranous layers (Fig. 2.34: diagram d, Fig. 2.39).
- The heterogeneous content, especially visible on the T2-weighted sequence, with appearance of small water bubbles within the silicone, called the sign of "salad oil"(Fig. 2.34: diagram e, Fig. 2.40).

ICR on MRI

- Linguine sign.
- Keyhole, noose or teardrop.
- Salad oil.

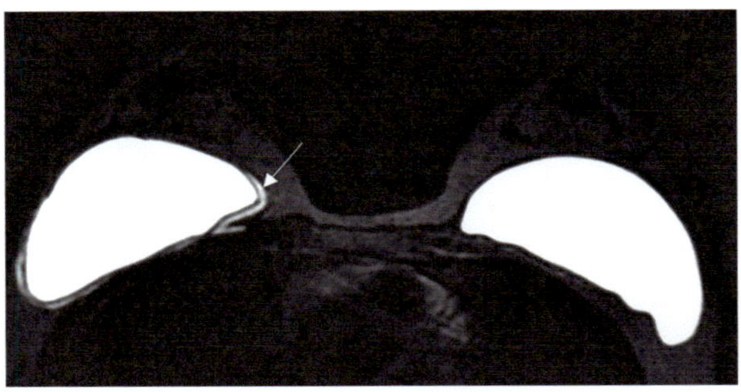

Fig. 2.38 Breast MRI "silicone only" sequence. Beginning ICR. On the right, silicone perspiration around the envelope without visible membranous floating. It is a very early intracapsular rupture

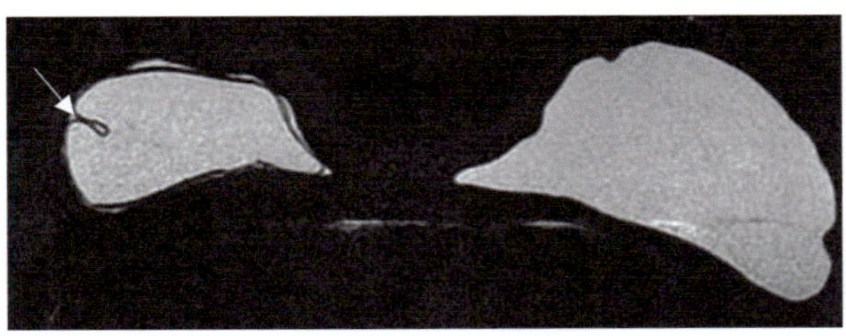

Fig. 2.39 Breast MRI "silicone only" sequence. ICR. On the right: "keyhole"appearance

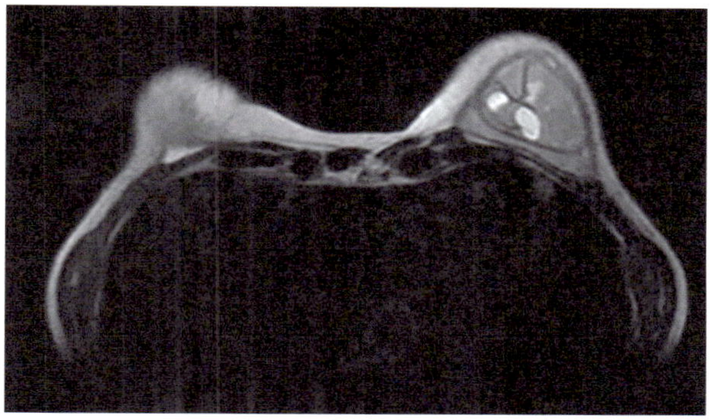

Fig. 2.40 Breast MRI T2-weighted sequence, without fat saturation. Advanced ICR. On the left, there is a heterogeneous content, with liquid bubbles within the silicone-filled implant, and a characteristic linguine sign

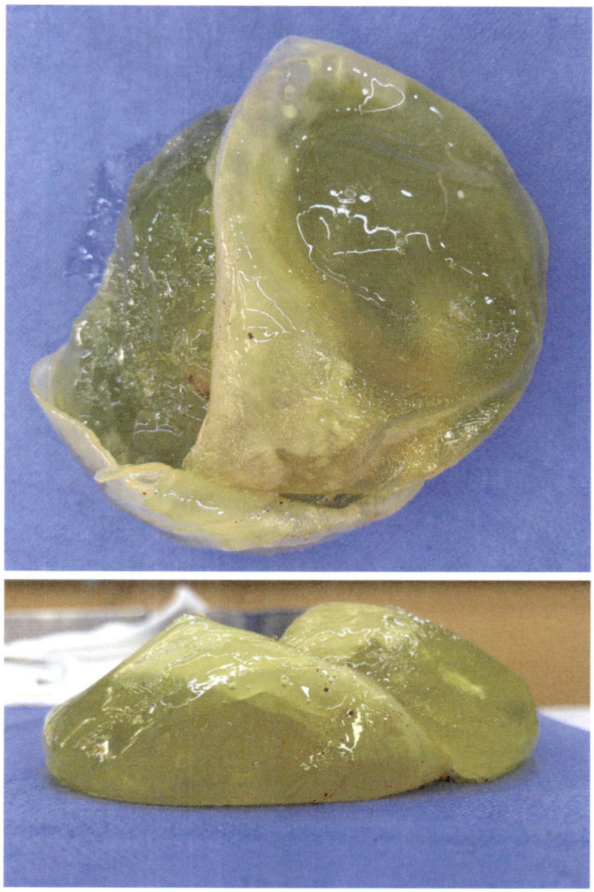

Fig. 2.41 Photo of a silicone-filled implant with ECR secondary to a violent trauma. The membrane is no longer continuous. A big hole can be seen

Extracapsular rupture (ECR).

It concerns all silicone-filled implants and occurs between 1 and 3 years after an intracapsular rupture or after a violent trauma [11] (Fig. 2.41). The implant is broken, and the silicone is outside the capsule, in the breast. The formed clusters are called siliconomas. They are generally peri-prosthetic, within the mammary gland. Their number and location should be specified in the radiological report for patient follow-up and for the plastic surgeon.

These can be palpable or asymptomatic. There is no overall loss of breast volume. This type of rupture can partially mask breast cancer. During the patient evaluation, it is important to know if the patient has a history of extracapsular rupture, with a prosthetic change, as there are often small siliconomas left even after cleaning, which can be misleading in imaging. They must be properly associated with the old rupture and not linked to the new intact implant.

Mammography

There are dense bands or dense clusters, around the implant or at a distance, related to the siliconomas. They can be associated with a deformation of the implant and all the signs of intracapsular rupture.

They are often associated with dense adenomegalies of the axilla, due to the ganglionic uptake of silicone [8].

The diagnosis on mammography is easier than that of the intracapsular rupture (Fig. 2.42 and 2.43a).

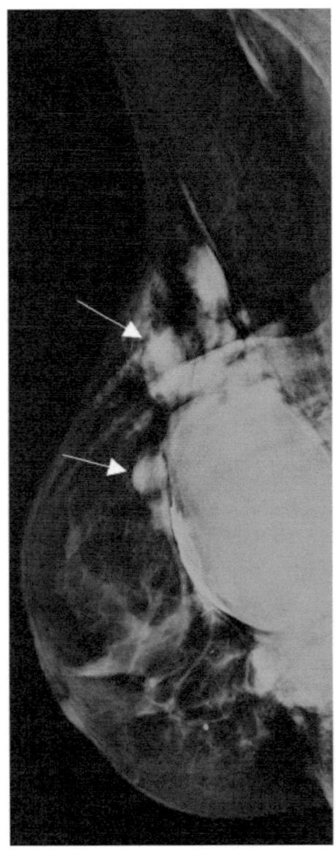

Fig. 2.42 Right MLO view. ECR; Numerous dense masses related to siliconomas, associated with a major deformation of the implant

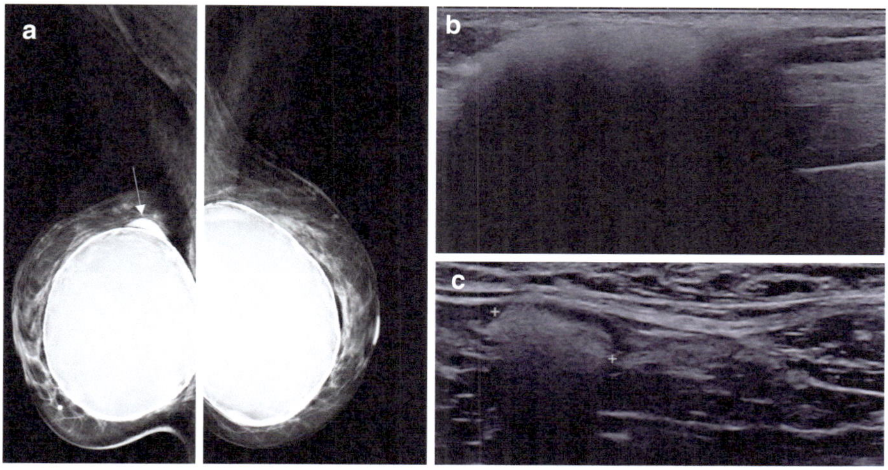

Fig. 2.43 Bilateral intracapsular rupture associated with an extracapsular rupture on the right. (**a**) Bilateral mammography MLO view. Periprothetic siliconoma at the right superior pole of the implant (white arrow). (**b**) Ultrasound image of the right breast. "Snowstorm"cluster outside the implant. (**c**) Right axillary ultrasound image. Ganglionic uptake of silicone in the axilla

Ultrasound

The appearance of extracapsular silicone is characteristic, in the form of hyperechoic masses with poorly defined contours known as "snowstorm", with posterior attenuation, which can be anywhere in the breast, but which are most often in contact with the implant [10] (Fig. 2.43b and 2.44).

The signs of intracapsular rupture are often associated.

The axilla should also be examined carefully for siliconic lymph nodes, even small ones (Fig. 2.43c).

> Do not confuse siliconomas from an old rupture with an extracapsular rupture. It is important to assess the condition of the capsulo-membranous complex and to correlate this with the woman's past surgical history. (Fig 2.44).

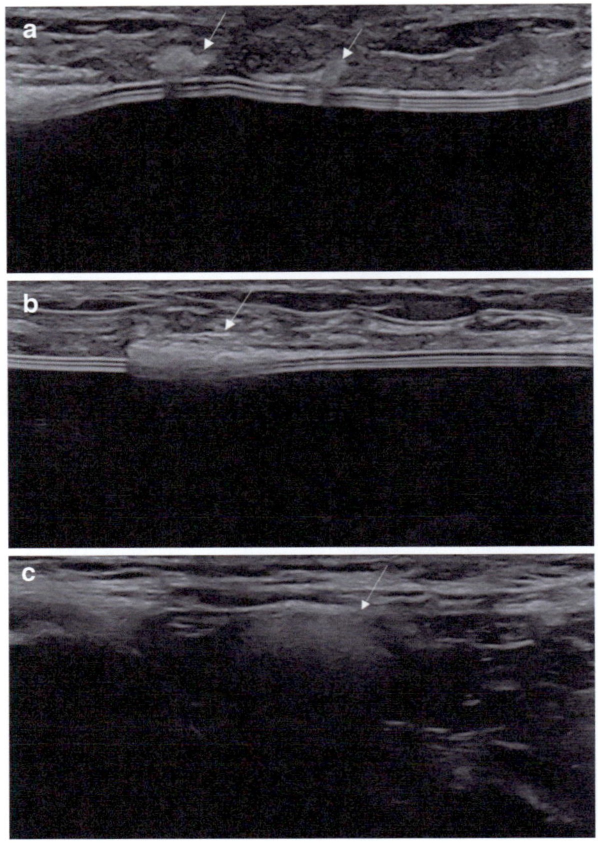

Fig. 2.44 Breast ultrasound of the right breast (a and b) and the right axilla (c). Sequelae of extracapsular rupture. Change of implants a few years ago, following an extracapsular rupture of the right breast implant. The current implant is intact. Small hyperechoic and attenuating siliconomas can be seen, attached to the implant as well as siliconic lymph nodes of the axillary region, all related to the old rupture. The capsulo-membranous complex is intact

MRI

Silicone is outside the implant, hyperintense on the WATER-STIR-weighted sequence and hypointense on the other sequences (Fig. 2.45).

The signs of ICR are often associated.

Imaging is interesting preoperatively to visualize the extent of the siliconoma and to have an overview.

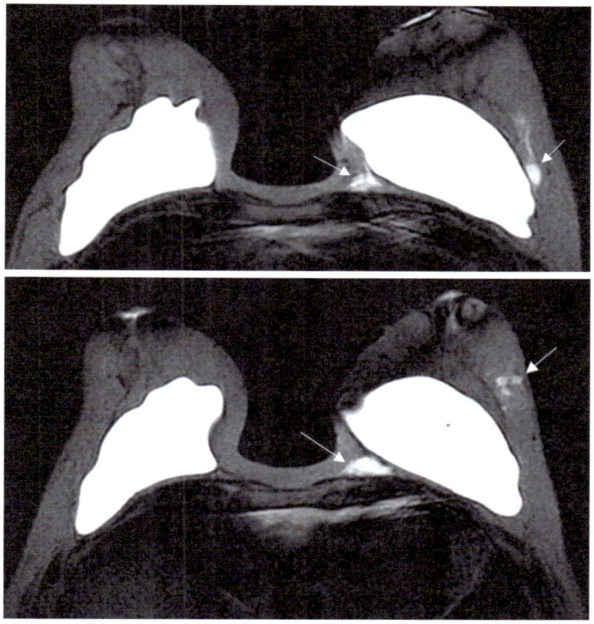

Fig. 2.45 Breast MRI WATER-STIR-weighted sequence "silicone only". Old ECR. The current implants are intact, but there are siliconomas on the left, due to an old rupture. Despite the cleaning by the surgeon during the prosthetic change (or simple extraction), there may still be small siliconomas around the capsule

The rupture of saline implants

It's a clinical diagnosis. Indeed, within a few hours, the implant and therefore the breast completely sag because the physiological saline is absorbed.

On mammography, as on ultrasound, a completely deflated implant is easily visualized (Fig. 2.46).

> MRI is not useful for diagnosis (Fig. 2.47).

Normally, extraction or replacement of the implant is recommended, but there are cases of patients who have kept their deflated implant for years in their breast without this causing a complication.

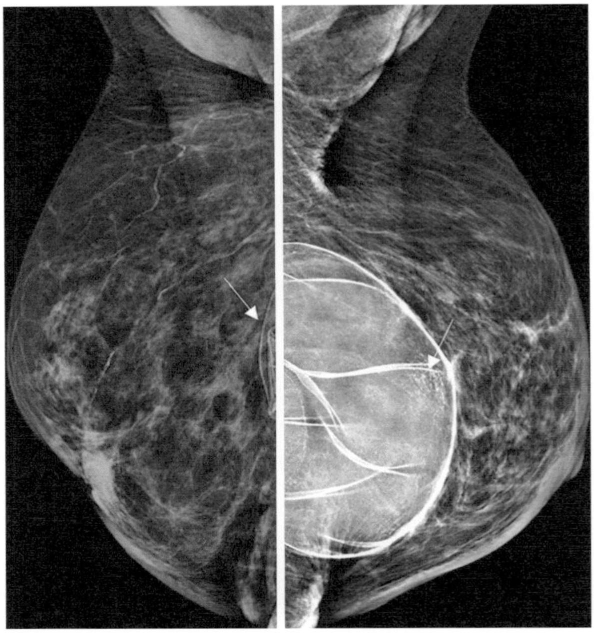

Fig. 2.46 Ruptured saline-filled implant. Bilateral mammography in MLO view. On the left, the saline implant is intact, easily recognizable because it is less dense than silicone. Note that there are fine parietal calcifications (arrow). On the right, deflated, it has lost its volume, and the membrane wall appears wrinkled, at the bottom of the prosthetic pocket, flattened by the pectoral muscle (arrow)

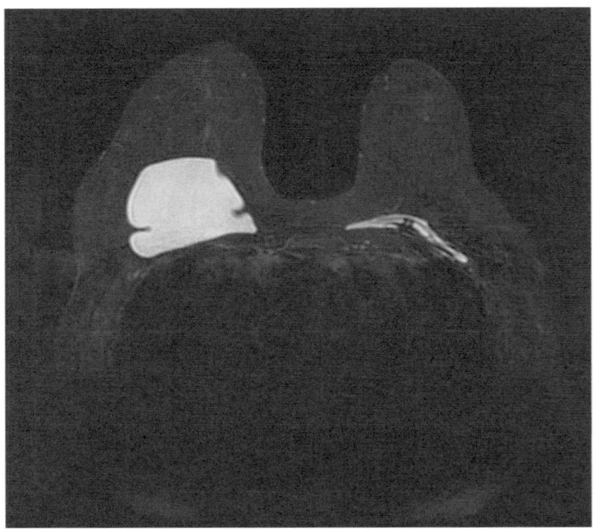

Fig. 2.47 Ruptured saline-filled implant. "T2 WATER" sequence breast MRI (fat signal saturation). MRI was performed, due to a high familial breast risk in the patient. The left saline implant left in place appears ruptured, with a wrinkled membrane

2.3.2 Capsular Contracture

It is the most common complication, and it is a clinical diagnosis [12]. It is a contracture of the capsule following an excessive inflammatory reaction, with tightening of the pocket and therefore of the implant. A peri-capsular fibrosis then appears.

The severity of capsular contracture is graded using the Baker classification (Table 2.2).

Capsular contracture occurs in 7% of cases when first put in place, on one or both breasts. In stages III and IV of Baker, the breast appears retracted and indurated, in excessive reaction to the foreign body that is the implant. It can occur early or later.

The origin is multifactorial (post-operative hematoma, autoimmune disease, tobacco...) [13]. It could be a subclinical bacterial infection on the surface of the prosthetic membrane. It occurs more frequently when the implant is located retroglandular rather than retropectoral. Macrotextured implants reduce this risk but cause other complications.

Imaging may be requested to rule out a differential or superimposed diagnosis.

In mammography: there may be a range of associated signs:

- A deformation, with a loss of the normal ovoid shape and a so-called "globular" implant (Fig. 2.48 and 2.49).

Table 2.2 Table of the Baker classification

Grade	Appearance	Palpability	Pain
I	Natural	Implant moves freely	No
II	Looks normal	Palpable firmness	No
III	Visible distortion	Firm and visible	Discomfort
IV	Abnormal	Tight and painful	Severe pain

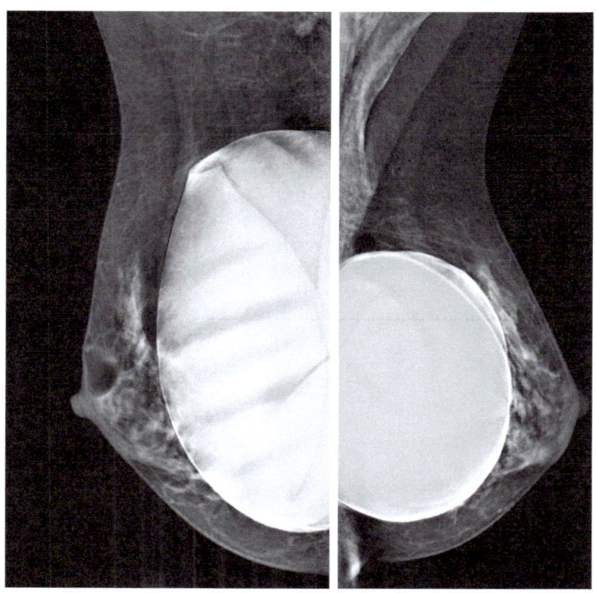

Fig. 2.48 Bilateral mammography in MLO view. Capsular contracture. Significant capsular contracture on the right causing a deformation of the implant visible in imaging. The diagnosis remains clinical

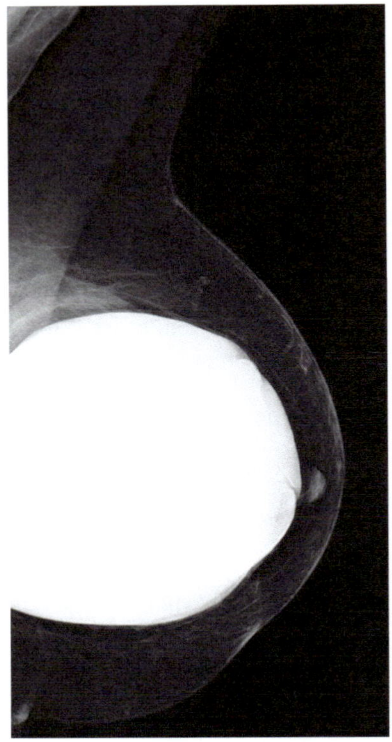

Fig. 2.49 Left MLO mammography. Capsular contracture. The implant appears deformed, typically globular

- An increase in the number of folds, however, it is difficult to evaluate this in practice, especially without priors for comparison.
- A reactive thickening of the capsule of more than 2 mm (a normal capsule has a thickness of about 1 mm) [14].

One may also observe the presence of thickened capsular tissue within the residual pocket following the removal of breast implants (Figs. 2.50 and 2.51). This tissue can be calcified or contain silicone if the removed implant was ruptured (Fig. 2.48).

In ultrasound and MRI: there may be:

- An increase in the number of folds.
- A reactive thickening of the capsule by more than 2 mm (Fig. 2.52).

Capsular Contracture: Clinical Diagnosis

– In imaging: +/−deformation of the implant, thickening of the capsule, increase in the number of folds.

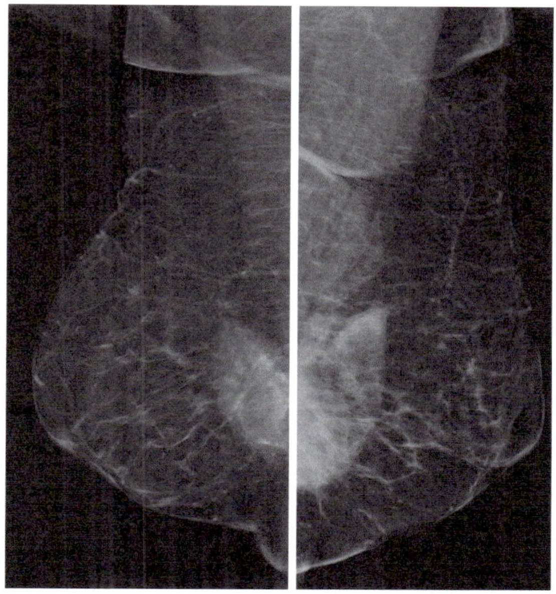

Fig. 2.50 Bilateral oblique mammography. Residual retroglandular shells. Non-pathological aspect with remaining capsule or scar tissue that can be left after implant extraction. We also visualize the fibrous retroareolar bands related to the mastopexy performed after extraction

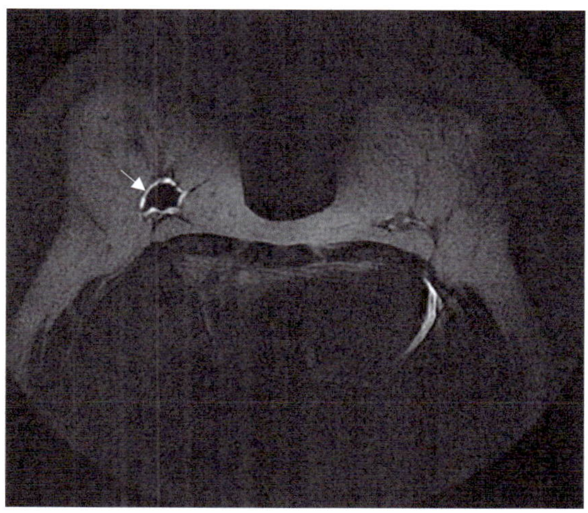

Fig. 2.51 Breast ultrasound. Capsular contracture. Thickening of the fibrous capsule by more than 2 mm

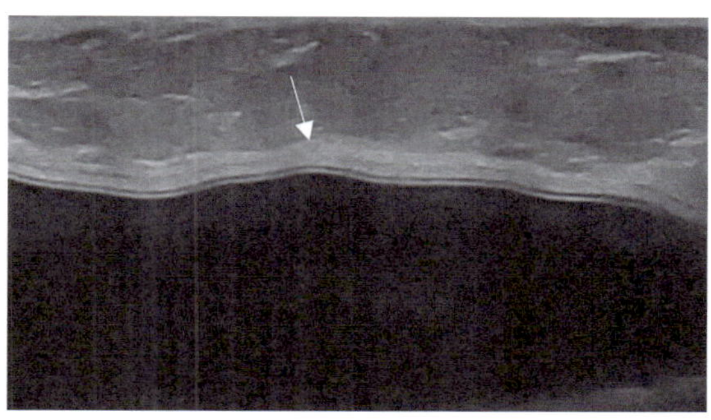

Fig. 2.52 Breast MRI. WATER-STIR sequence "silicone only". Residual shells after prosthetic extraction. The shells appear as a fibrous area in relation to the old prosthetic sites. There is also residual silicone around the shell on the right (arrow)

2.3.3 Seroma Formation

Physiologically, there is a minimal peri-implant fluid. It often can be encountered between the prosthetic folds.

If it is more significant, it can be a sign of:

- An infection (especially early post-operative), which requires antibiotic treatment or even removal of the implant.
- An idiopathic inflammatory episode (Fig. 2.53), this can be quickly resolved under anti-inflammatory treatment or turn into chronic seroma.
- Or finally, be the first sign of anaplastic large cell lymphoma (ALCL).

Mammography reveals a dense peri-prosthetic band (Fig. 2.53a).

Ultrasound confirms the existence of the liquid effusion (Fig. 2.53b, c), sometimes dense.

MRI, if performed, also shows the peri-prosthetic fluid (Fig. 2.54), provides an overview, and identifies a possible underlying etiology (Fig. 2.55).

Imaging allows us to quantify the effusion.

A needle aspiration can be performed, especially for diagnostic purposes, for example in case of suspicion of ALCL.

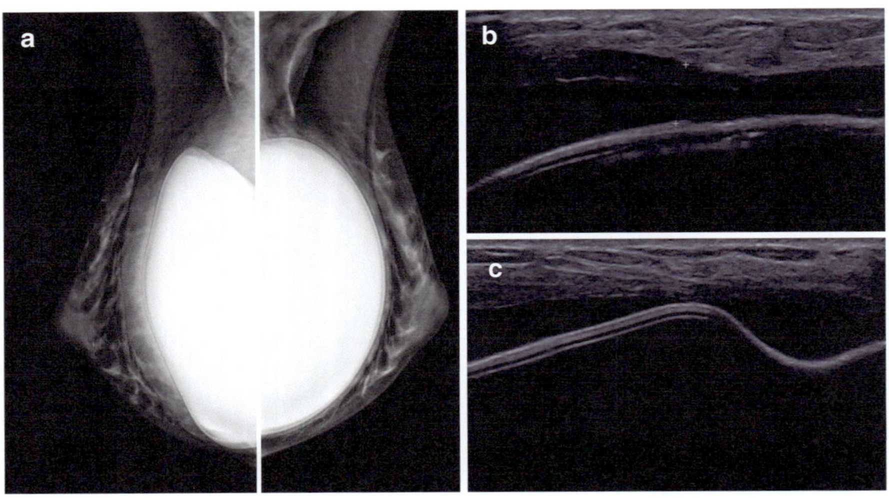

Fig. 2.53 Bilateral mammography in MLO view (**a**) and two ultrasound images of the right breast (**b**, **c**). Inflammatory peri-prosthetic effusion. Presence of a right peri-prosthetic effusion appearing as a hyperdense peri-prosthetic band on mammography and an anechoic peri-prosthetic fluid on ultrasound. The implant is intact. MRI is not indicated. The episode spontaneously resolved with anti-inflammatory treatment

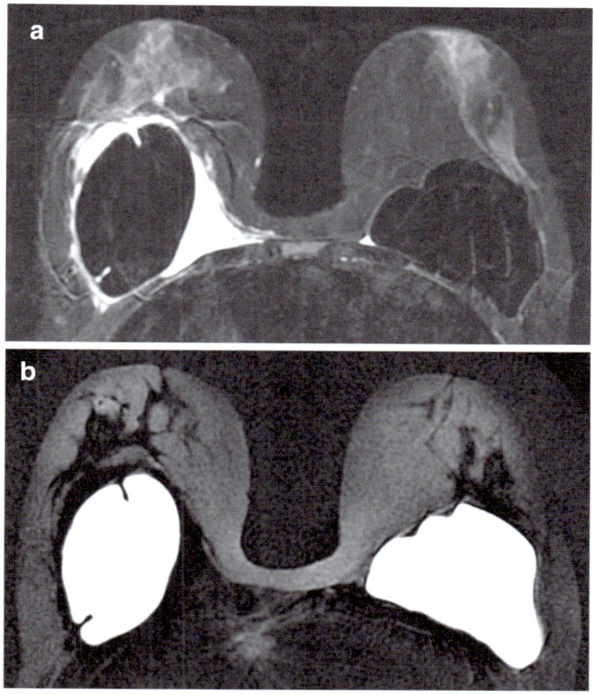

Fig. 2.54 MRI in T2 WATER sequence (with fat saturation) (**a**) and "silicone only" sequence (**b**). Effusion peri-prosthetic inflammatory liquid effusion with high signal intensity on T2-weighted imaging. (arrow). On the WATER-STIR sequence, the effusion is hypointense, purely liquid, whereas the silicone of the implants appears very hyperintense. Note the artifacts on the T2-WATER sequence, due to the patient's respiratory movements

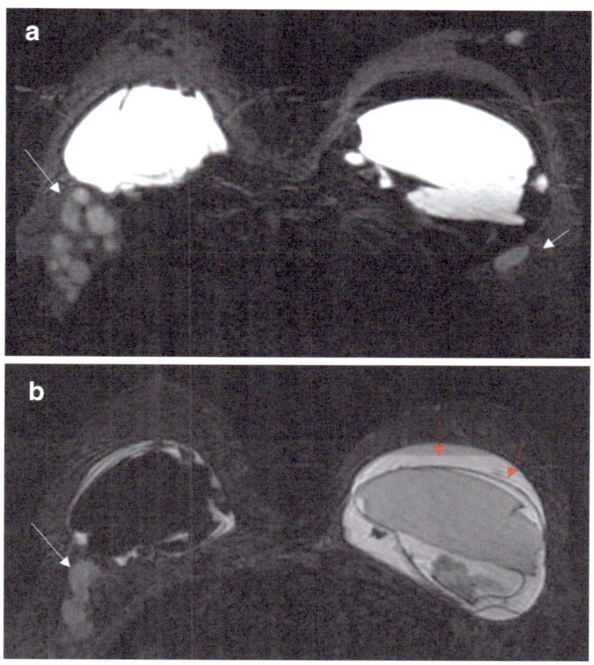

Fig. 2.55 Breast MRI. Periprosthetic effusion and rupture. (**a**) "Silicone only" sequence and (**b**) T2 sequence with fat signal saturation. Intracapsular rupture with "linguine sign" on the left, periprosthetic effusion in T2 hypersignal especially marked on the left (red arrows), and bilateral axillary silicone nodes (white arrows)

2.3.4 Rotation

There are two types of rotation [15]:

In both cases, it is an implant that is no longer positioned as it was initially placed.

- The first type is rotation between the hourly rays and concerns exclusively the anatomical implants: We speak classically of rotation, when the patient or the clinician notes clinically an asymmetry or a deformation of the contours. In fact, it exists a rotation in 27% of cases but which is perceptible clinically only in 5% of cases. The diagnosis is made by ultrasound by visualizing the raised markers on the prosthetic membrane (bulges), in the form of small rounded buttons or edge depending on the brands, which are no longer positioned between the rays of 5 o'clock and 7 o'clock (Figs. 2.56 and 2.57).

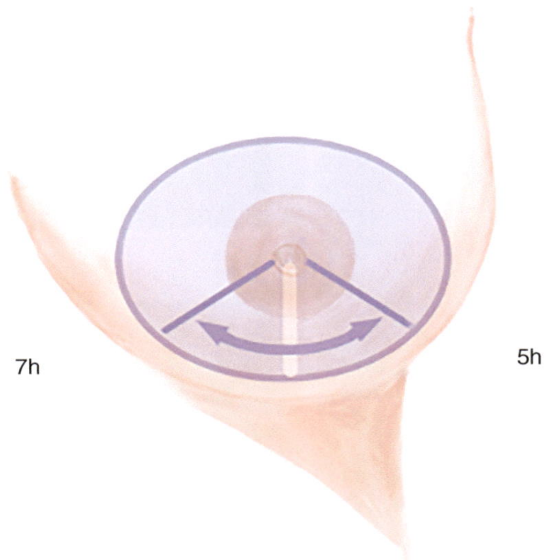

Fig. 2.56 Diagram of a breast with hourly rays. The markers (dotted lines) must be positioned between the rays of 5 h and 7 h, otherwise it is a rotation. Here, they are at the 6 O'clock position

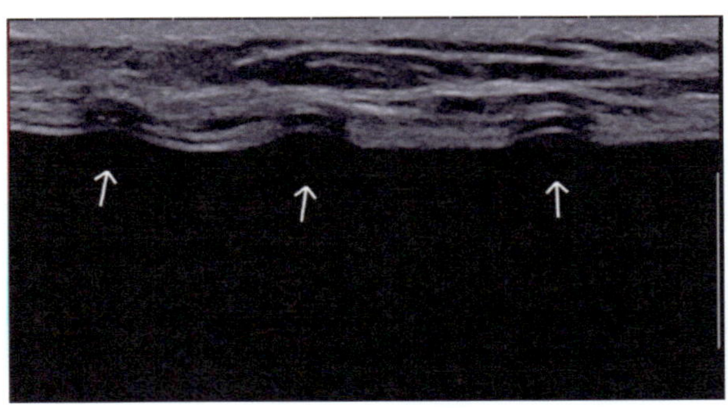

Fig. 2.57 Breast ultrasound. Rotation. Ultrasound image on the right external quadrants showing the three displaced anatomical markers, located outside the hourly rays 5–7 h

Sometimes, the markers are visible at mammography (Fig. 2.18), but the exact positioning is difficult to evaluate with this technique. One can however see the deformation and the asymmetry compared to the contralateral side, when the rotation is important. This remains very rare (Fig. 2.58).

- The second type of rotation is more anecdotal: it is a complete reversal of the implant, with the posterior wall of the implant ending up in front.

In imaging, one can then see the occlusion patch in the anterior position (Figs. 2.59 and 2.60). Generally, there is no clinical consequence. MRI is not useful for diagnosis of this complication.

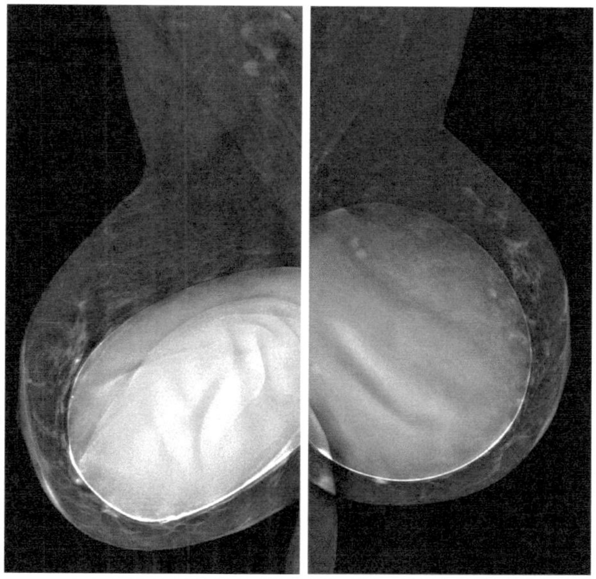

Fig. 2.58 Bilateral mammography in MLO View. Rotation. Anatomical silicone-filled implant in retroglandular position. The right implant appears turned, with a deformation and an asymmetry compared to the left side

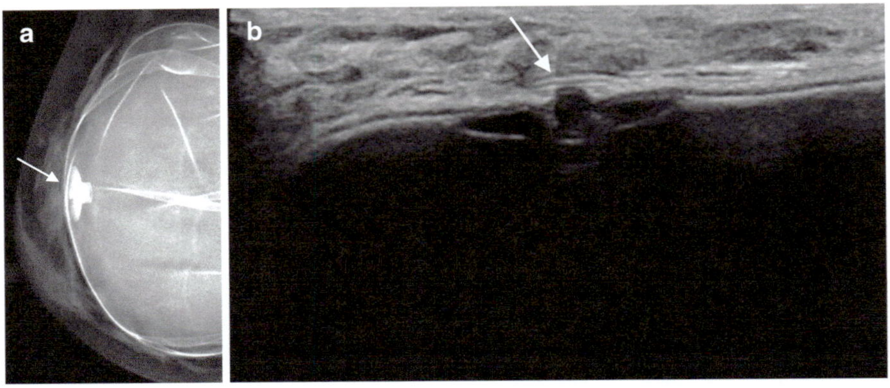

Fig. 2.59 Rotation. (**a**) Right mammography in MLO View. (**b**) Ultrasound image of the same breast. Round saline implant turned over, with posterior occlusion patch visualized in front (arrow), both on the mammography image and on the ultrasound

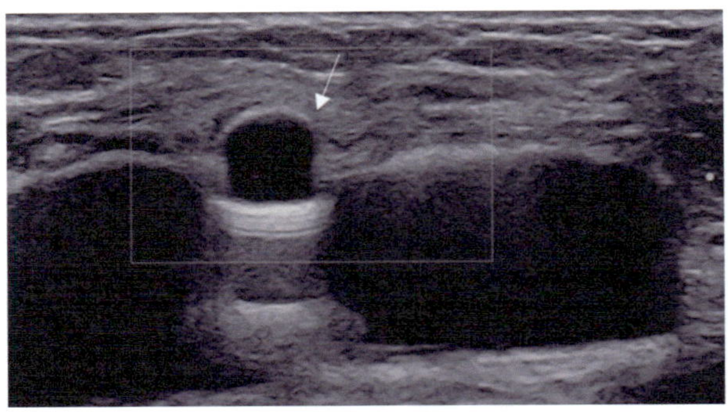

Fig. 2.60 Breast ultrasound. Rotation. Round saline implant turned over in the antero-posterior direction. We observe the occlusion patch with a plug in the anterior position (arrow)

2.3.5 Herniation

Herniation is rarely described.

The envelope of the implant is more or less extensible and elastic. Over time, it can form herniation when silicone gel or saline, push out through a weak spot of the capsule. These herniations, which are exacerbated by muscle compression when the implant is retropectoral, are sometimes caused by trauma, sometimes spontaneous. They can range from a frank herniation with a voluminous expansion, to a simple bulge in the prosthetic contour. In imaging, it can be a simple lobulation of the implant contour or a diverticular type of deformation (Fig. 2.61).

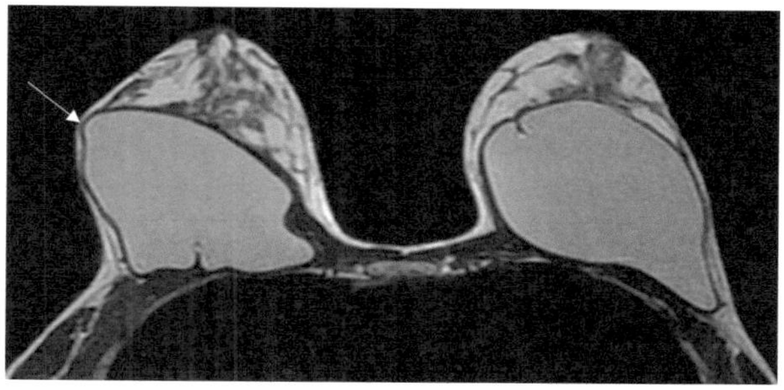

Fig. 2.61 T2-weighted sequence breast MRI without fat saturation. Implant herniation. On the right, there is a weak spot of the capsule with herniation of the implant externally and a bulging aspect, palpable (arrow)

2.3.6 Silicone Lymphadenopathy

It appears in case of rupture or even simply with the age of the implant, due to a lymphatic drainage of silicone. However, this latter phenomenon is infrequent and especially reported for the old implants and PIP implants (poor quality porous membrane), less common for the new generations of implants.

It can be seen in the axillary or internal mammary area. It does not require specific treatment.

The mammography shows dense adenomegalies in the axilla (Fig. 2.62a).

The ultrasound finds hyperechoic and attenuating lymph nodes, in a "snowstorm"pattern like for siliconoma of the breast. They can be visualized in the axilla or along the internal mammary chain (Fig. 2.62b, c).

The MRI also finds the axillary or internal mammary lymph nodes, filled with silicone, clearly visible on the "silicone only" sequence, in hypersignal (Fig. 2.63).

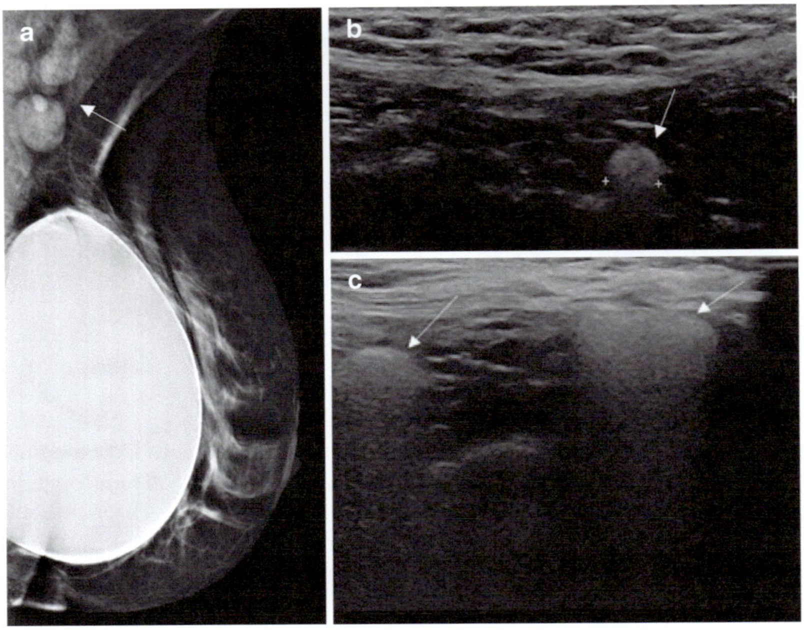

Fig. 2.62 Silicone lymphadenopathy. Left mammography MLO view (**a**). Breast ultrasound image on the axilla (**b**, **c**). Intact retropectoral silicone implant, with a homolateral axillary lymph node uptake, in the form of dense adenomegalies on mammography (**a**). On ultrasound, we confirm the siliconic content of the lymph nodes which appear hyperechoic and attenuating, in a "snowstorm" (**b**, **c**)

Fig. 2.63 Breast MRI. Silicone lymphadenopathy. Two MRI slices in "silicone only" sequence showing bilateral axillary and internal mammary siliconic lymph nodes in hypersignal, with intact implants

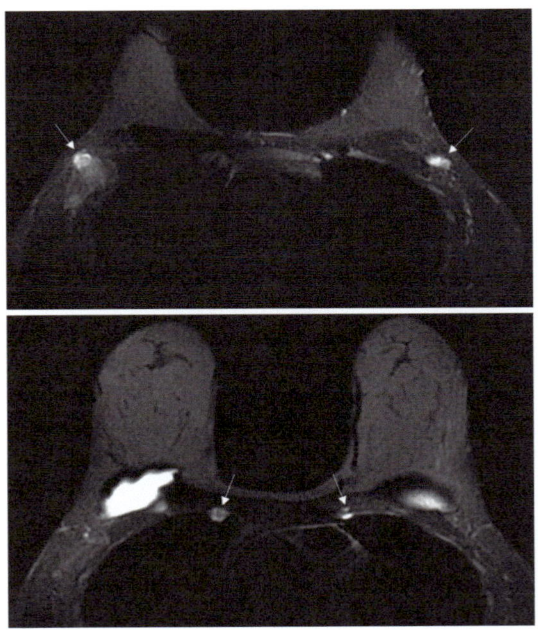

2.3.7 Anaplastic Large Cell Lymphoma (ALCL)

Textured implants were developed in the 2000s (2002 in France) to create a local inflammation, with white blood cells eliminating the biofilm around the implant, in opposition to smooth implants which were responsible for capsular contracture in 10–15% of cases (the leading cause of reoperation). This has reduced the incidence to about 5%.

The first cases of lymphomas were noted in 2009, between 1 and 25 years after the placement (on average 7 years) [16]. It is a lymphoma anaplastic large cell associated with breast implants (ALCL-BI), linked to the textured membrane of the implants (as well as a bacterial contamination and a genetic predisposition) [17, 18]. The incidence is estimated at 1/30,000 patients [19]. There are no confirmed cases with smooth implants.

It is mainly found with macro-textured implants, with 1 case out of 2200 patients, which is more than the micro-textured or nano-textured implants.

Clinically, in 90% of cases, it presents with a moderate to high abundance of rapid onset effusion, most often with an increase in breast volume and pain.

Mammography and ultrasound show:

- A peri-prosthetic effusion of varying importance and density (Fig. 2.64a).
- +/− associated masses or tissue thickening, vascularized in doppler ultrasound (Fig. 2.64b).

It is interesting to complete the assessment with a CT scan or an injected MRI to visualize the extent of the lesions, or even the pectoral extension (Fig. 2.64c).

The diagnosis is made by needle aspiration of the liquid with cytology and specific search for the CD30 membrane antigen on the cell surface. The double pathological reading is essential to ensure an accurate and reliable diagnosis of lymphoma associated with breast implants, due to its complexity and the need for specialized expertise.

Four stages are defined: IA when malignant cells are exclusively found within the effusion, IB on the capsular surface, IC in the capsule, IIA if the capsule is breached. We talk about stages IIB, III, IV, in case of lymph node invasion and distant organ involvement but they are much rarer.

In 80% of cases, the removal of the implant and its capsule (capsulectomy) are the only treatment, with an excellent prognosis (Fig. 2.65).

In conclusion, within the specialized domain of breast implant imaging, it is imperative for radiologists to be well-versed in both the indications for preoperative and postoperative imaging, and to be familiar with the expected post-surgical appearances as well as potential misleading signs. Mastery of these elements is crucial for minimizing unnecessary imaging procedures without compromising diagnostic accuracy. By optimizing imaging strategies, radiologists can ensure efficient use of resources while maintaining the highest standard of patient care.

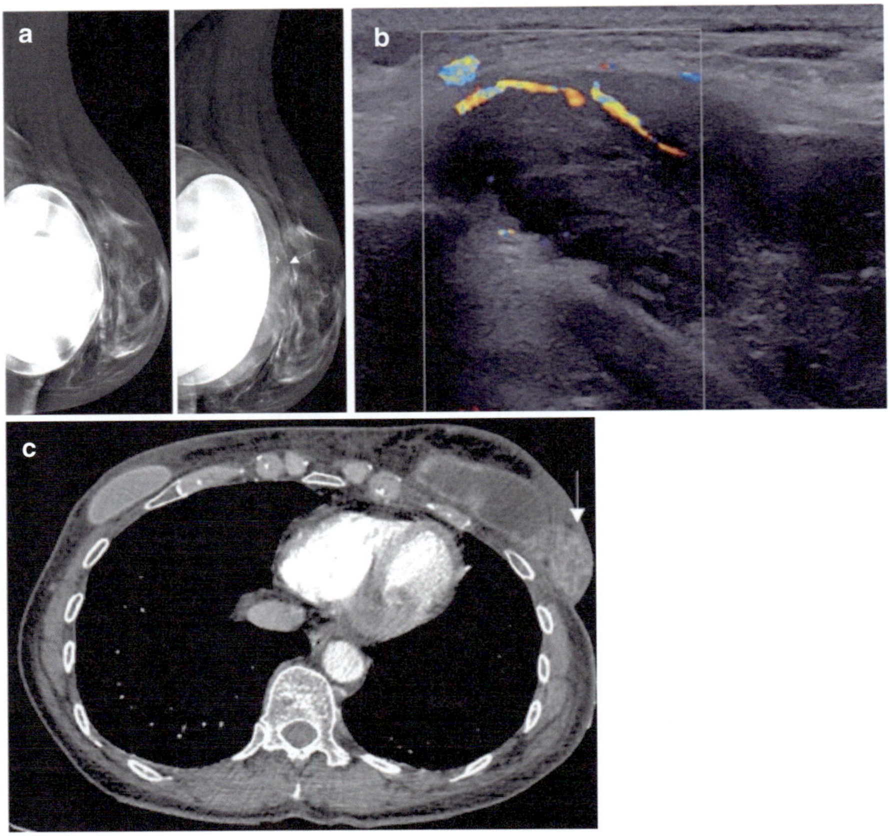

Fig. 2.64 ALCL-BI. (**a**) Left MLO mammograms at 8-month intervals. Mammograms in the same patient, returned at 8-month intervals due to a painful and rapid increase in breast volume. We note the appearance of a peri-prosthetic effusion. (**b**) Doppler-color ultrasound of the left breast. Vascularization of a tissue portion within the heterogeneous effusion. The analysis of the fluid by needle aspiration with specific search for the CD30 membrane antigen on the cell surface, confirms the diagnosis of anaplastic large cell lymphoma. (**c**) Axial slice of injected thoracic CT scan. CT scan performed after simple prosthetic explantation. On the left, there is a residual collection, but especially a contrast-enhancing tissue portion, which requires a surgical revision with wide excision

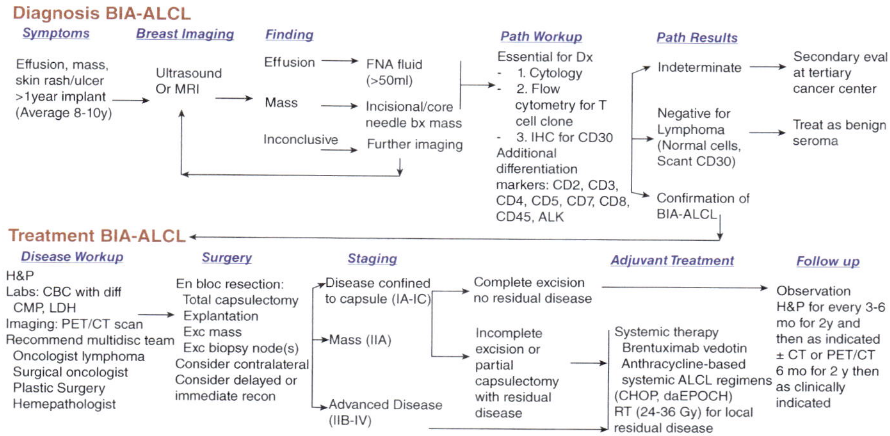

Fig. 2.65 ALCL-BI Table. 2019 NCCN Consensus guidelines on the Diagnosis and Treatment of Breast Implant-Associated Anaplastic Large Cell Lymphoma (BIA-ALCL)

References

1. Chao A, Garza R 3rd, Povoski SP. A review of the use of silicone implants in breast surgery. Expert Rev Med Devices. 2016;13(2):143–56.
2. Handel N, Silverstein MJ. Breast cancer diagnosis and prognosis in augmented women. Plast Reconstr Surg. 2006;118(3):587–93; discussion 594–6
3. Mimoun M, et al. A 10-year follow-up experience of 383 patients with bilateral smooth inflatable breast implants filled with saline solution. Aesth Plast Surg. 2020;44(2):330–8.
4. Expert Panel ON Breast I, et al. ACR appropriateness criteria® for breast implant evaluation. J Am Coll Radiol. 2018;15(5S):S13–25.
5. Carloni R, et al. Preoperative imaging prior to breast reconstruction surgery: benchmarking bringing together radiologists and plastic surgeons. Proposed guidelines. Ann Chir Plast Esthet. 2014;59(2):e13–9.
6. Stivala, et al. Efficacy of ultrasound, mammography, and magnetic resonance imaging in detecting breast implant rupture: a retrospective study of 175 reconstructive and aesthetic subpectoral breast augmentation cases. J Plast Reconstr Aesthet Surg. 2017;70(11):1520–6.
7. Stoblen F, Rezai M, Akummel S. Imaging in patients with breast implants results of the first international breast (implant) conference 2009. Insights Imaging. 2010;1(2):93–7.
8. Georgieva M, et al. Imaging of breast implant and implant-associated complications: capsular contracture and intra or extracapsular rupture. Clin Hemorheol Microcirc. 2020;76(2):221–31.
9. Seiler SJ, et al. Multimodality imaging-based evaluation of single-lumen silicone breast implants for rupture. Radiographics. 2017;37(2):366–82.
10. Rochira D, et al. Longitudinal ultrasound study of breast implant rupture over a six-year interval. Ann Plast Surg. 2016;76(2):150–4.
11. Cj C, et al. FDA breast implant Postapproval studies: long-term outcomes in 99,993 patients. Ann Surg. 2019;269(1):30–6.
12. Bachour Y, Ritt M. Risk factors for developing capsular contracture in women after breast implant surgery: a systematic review of the literature. J Plast Reconstr Aesthet Surg. 2018;71(11):e68.

13. Virden CP, et al. Subclinical infection of the silicone breast implant surface as a possible cause of capsular contracture. Aesth Plast Surg. 2020;44(4):1141–7.
14. Gossner J. Sonography in capsular contracture after breast augmentation: value of established criteria, new techniques and directions for research. J Ultrasound. 2017;20(1):87–9.
15. Sieber DA, et al. Clinical Evaluation of Shaped gel Breast Implant Rotation using high-Resolution ultrasound. Aesthet Surg J. 2017;37(3):290–6.
16. Groth AK, Graf R. Correction to: breast implant-associated anaplastic large cell lymphoma (BIA-ALCL) and the textured breast implant crisis. Aesthetic Plast Surg. 2020;44(5):1951.
17. Turton P, et al. UK guidelines on the diagnosis and treatment of breast implant-associated anaplastic large cell lymphoma (BIA-ALCL) on behalf of the medicines and healthcare products regulatory agency (MHRA) plastic, reconstructive and aesthetic surgery expert advisory group (PRASEAg). Eur J Surg Oncol. 2021;47(2):199–210.
18. Mb NAVA, et al. Is breast implant associated-anaplastic large cell lymphoma linked to textured implants? Aesth Plast Surg. 2021;45:2593.
19. Clemens MW, Jacobsen ED, Horwitz SM. NCCN consensus guidelines on the diagnosis and treatment of breast implant-associated anaplastic large cell lymphoma (BIA-ALCL). Aesthet Surg J. 2019;39(Suppl_1):S3–S13.

Breast Reduction and Mastopexy

3

Contents

3.1 Surgical Techniques

Breast reduction surgery, which involves a reduction in glandular, fatty, and skin volume, and reshaping at the same time, is performed in cases of hypertrophy [1], malformation, or for symmetrization after conservative contralateral treatment. The surgeon can make three types of scars [2]:

- A peri-areolar scar (Fig. 3.1a).
- A peri-areolar and vertical scar (from the areola to the submammary fold) (Fig. 3.1b).
- Or most often, a peri-areolar, vertical, and horizontal scar from the submammary fold, known as "inverted T"or "anchor" (Fig. 3.1c) with a higher repositioning of the areolo-mammary plate, sometimes a reduction in its size, and a harmonious distribution of the gland with a skin draping [3].

Mastopexy or breast lift, aims to lift the breast, without reducing its volume, but by removing the excess skin. The scars are the same as for breast reduction, even if the peri-areolar scar *(round block)* is reserved for very moderate ptosis [4].

S. Cohen-Zarade, *Imaging of Plastic Surgery of the Breast and Other Implants*,
https://doi.org/10.1007/978-3-031-64159-6_3

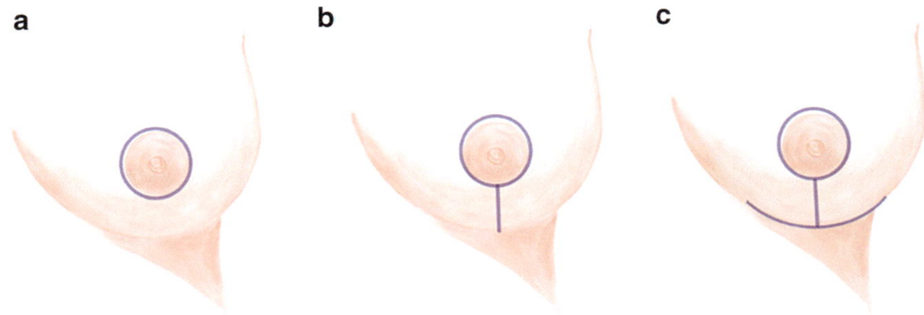

Fig. 3.1 Mastopexy scar diagrams; (**a**) peri-areolar (round *block*); (**b**) peri-areolar and vertical; (**c**) “inverted T“

The result should lead to a breast with fullness in the lower quadrants, and an areola well-centered on the volume, oriented horizontally or slightly upwards.

Mastopexy can be combined with the placement of an implant if the breast has been “emptied” following a pregnancy, breastfeeding, or significant weight loss, or if the breast volume is insufficient.

3.2 Imaging Protocol

The standard pre-surgical assessment includes a mammogram with two 2D views (front and oblique), a tomosynthesis acquisition, and an ultrasound depending on the breast density [5, 6].

Any lesion classified as ACR4, ACR5 or even ACR3 must be biopsied for histological analysis, before surgery [7, 8].

There is no formal consensus to date, but most surgeons prefer the mammography to be 6 months to 1 year old before the intervention [9].

The age of realization is mandatory after 40 years. Between 30 and 40 years, an ultrasound is performed and almost always a single MLO view of each breast, looking for microcalcifications.

Indeed, finding a cancer postoperatively (especially on the operative reduction piece) prevents the patient from benefiting from a conservative treatment, due to the lack of information on the initial location of the lesion.

The follow-up is identical to that of the general population [5]. The risk of developing breast cancer is the same in patients who have undergone a mastopexy compared to others.

There is no control to be carried out in the immediate postoperative period.

The MRI: It is not recommended to perform an MRI as a pre-operative measure or for routine monitoring of patients who have previously undergone a mastopexy.

Imaging Protocol

- Preoperative imaging conducted between 6 months to 1 year prior to the procedure.
- Follow-up identical to that of the general population.
- MRI not recommended in the preoperative assessment or for follow-up.

3.3 Imaging Appearances

After mastopexy, there is a non-pathological aspect, which must be known to avoid interpretation errors. Complications are rare, occurring in the immediate post-operative period, and rarely requiring imaging (hematoma, infection…).

The clinical examination should not be forgotten, including the examination of scars on the skin, to identify the surgical technique used.

3.3.1 Mammography

The first mammogram performed after intervention is very useful because it serves as a new reference for comparison during follow-ups [5]. It typically shows [10]:

- Thin fibrous retractile scars retroareolar and in the lower quadrants (Figs. 3.2 and 3.3), forming thin dense linear bands, concave upwards.
- A modification of the architecture of the mammary gland, which can sometimes hinder interpretation. Indeed, after reduction, the classic distribution of glandular tissue is modified, with a more central topographic location in the breast volume and a loss of the axillary extension. As a result, there is a global increase in breast density (Fig. 3.4).
- Round retroareolar microcalcifications, sometimes with a clear center, vertically arranged (Figs. 3.5 and 3.6).
- A smooth thickening of the nipple-areolar complex or of the skin (Figs. 3.2 and 3.3).
- Cutaneous calcifications, more or less dense (Figs. 3.5 and 3.6).
- Occasionally, rounded masses indicative of Fat necrosis or oil cysts may be present, characterized by a distinct central clarity and delicate boundaries, situated along the line of the surgical incision. These are associated with the surgical injury and subsequent necrosis of adipose cells. With time, the walls of these cysts may become calcified [11] (Fig. 3.7).

Mammographic Appearances

- Fibrous retractile scars.
- Modification of the architecture of the mammary gland.
- Retroareolar microcalcifications.
- Thickening of the nipple-areolar complex.
- Cutaneous calcifications.
- Fat necrosis.

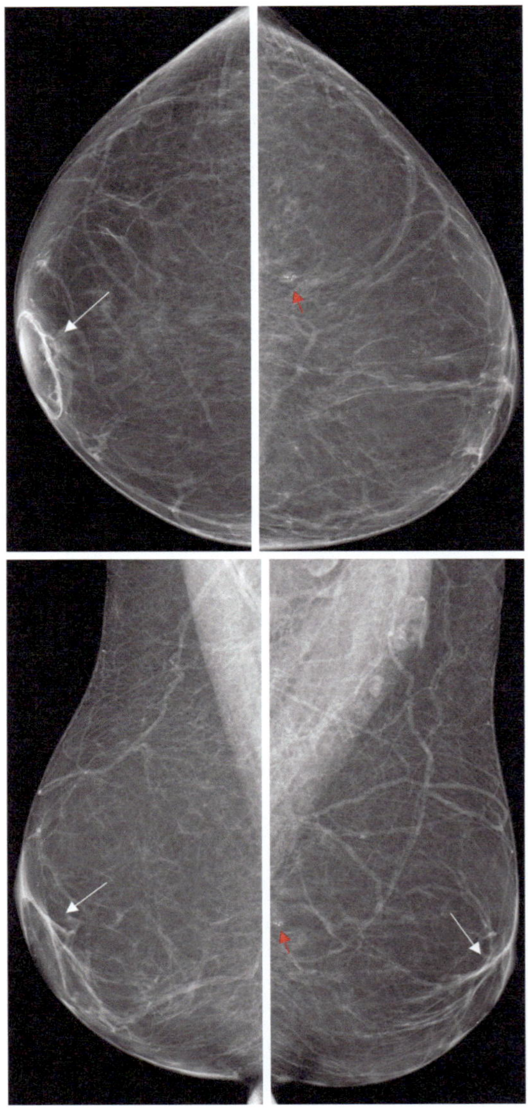

Fig. 3.2 Bilateral mammography. Breast reduction. Breasts with predominantly fatty tissue (Category A) according to the BI-RADS classification. There are retroareolar fibrous bands, especially marked on the CC view (arrows). There is also a thickening of the nipple-areolar complex. Notice a small calcified fibroadenoma at the junction of the left outer quadrants (red arrow)

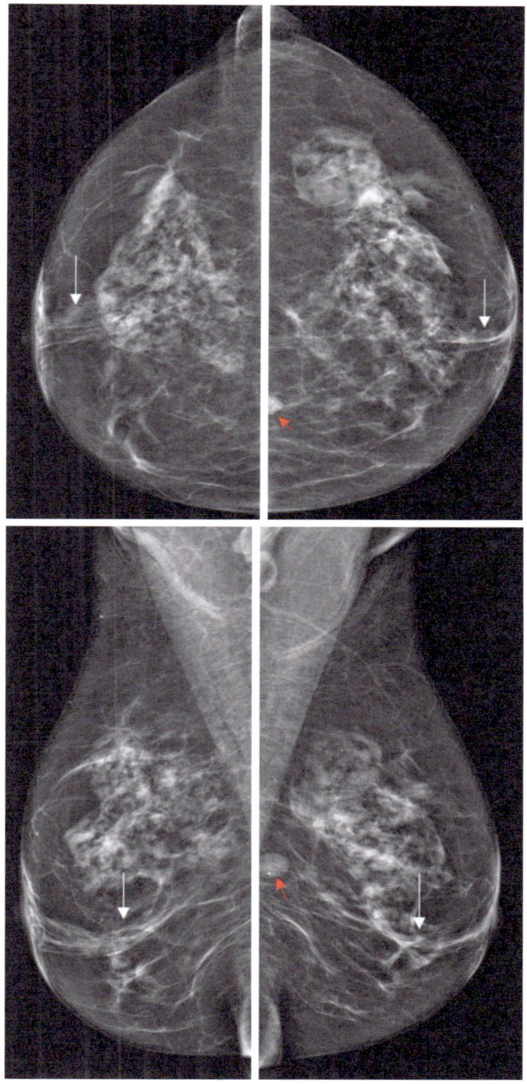

Fig. 3.3 Bilateral mammography. Breast reduction. Breasts with predominantly glandular tissue (Category C) according to the BI-RADS classification. Retroareolar fibrous bands, concave upwards (white arrows) on all views and redistribution of the mammary gland. There is also a thickening of the nipple-areolar complex. Note an upper-inner left cyst (red arrow)

One must remain vigilant for the study of the mammary parenchyma and not hesitate to perform additional views such as localized compression, magnified, localized compression in tomosynthesis, to identify a lesion within a denser parenchyma and scars (Figs. 3.8, 3.9 and 3.10).

An implant can be put in place in association with the mastopexy. The analysis and the semiology remain the same, with study of the implant and study of the breast parenchyma considering the usual aspects of the mastopexy (Figs. 3.11 and 3.12).

Stereotactic macrobiopsy or by tomosynthesis, can be performed in the same way as without a history of mastopexy.

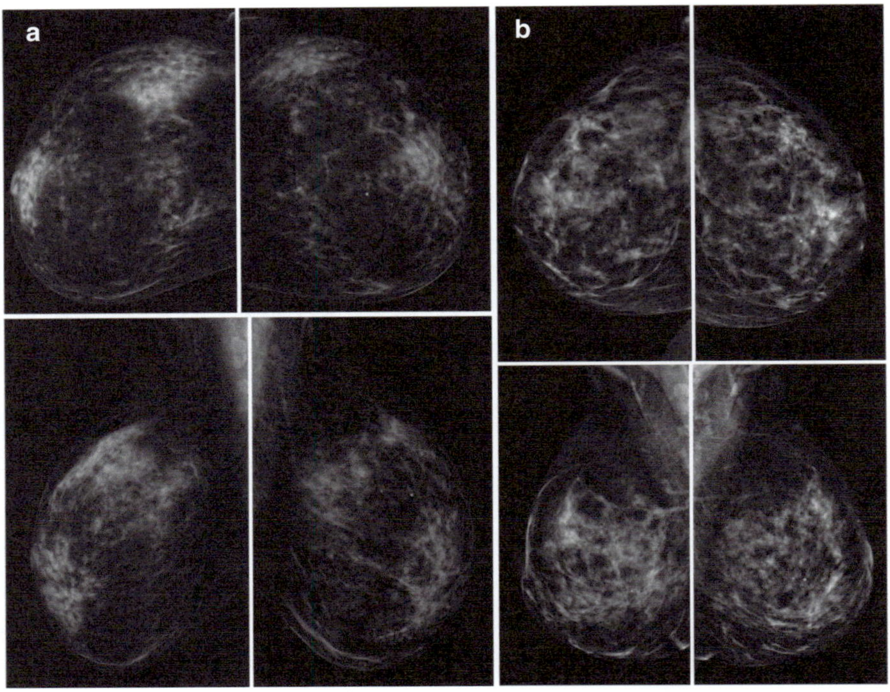

Fig. 3.4 Bilateral mammography before and after breast reduction. (**a**) Bilateral mammography before breast reduction. (**b**) Bilateral mammography 2 years after breast reduction. Volume reduction with a global increase in breast density and a more central distribution of the gland. There are thin retroareolar scar bands not hindering interpretation

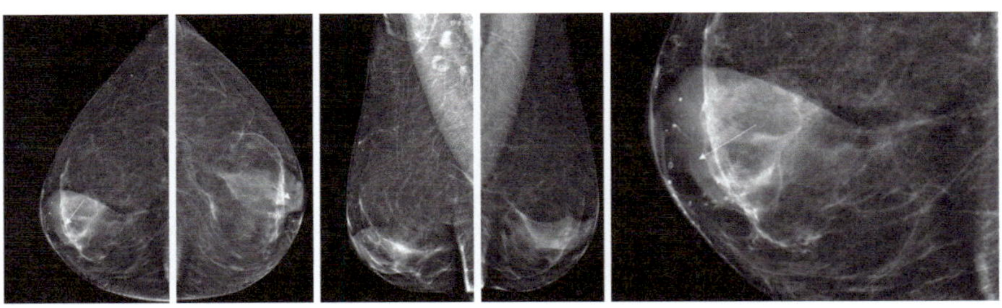

Fig. 3.5 Bilateral mammography after mastopexy. CC and MLO views, with zoom on the right CC view. Lucent-centered retroareolar and cutaneous calcifications are clearly visible

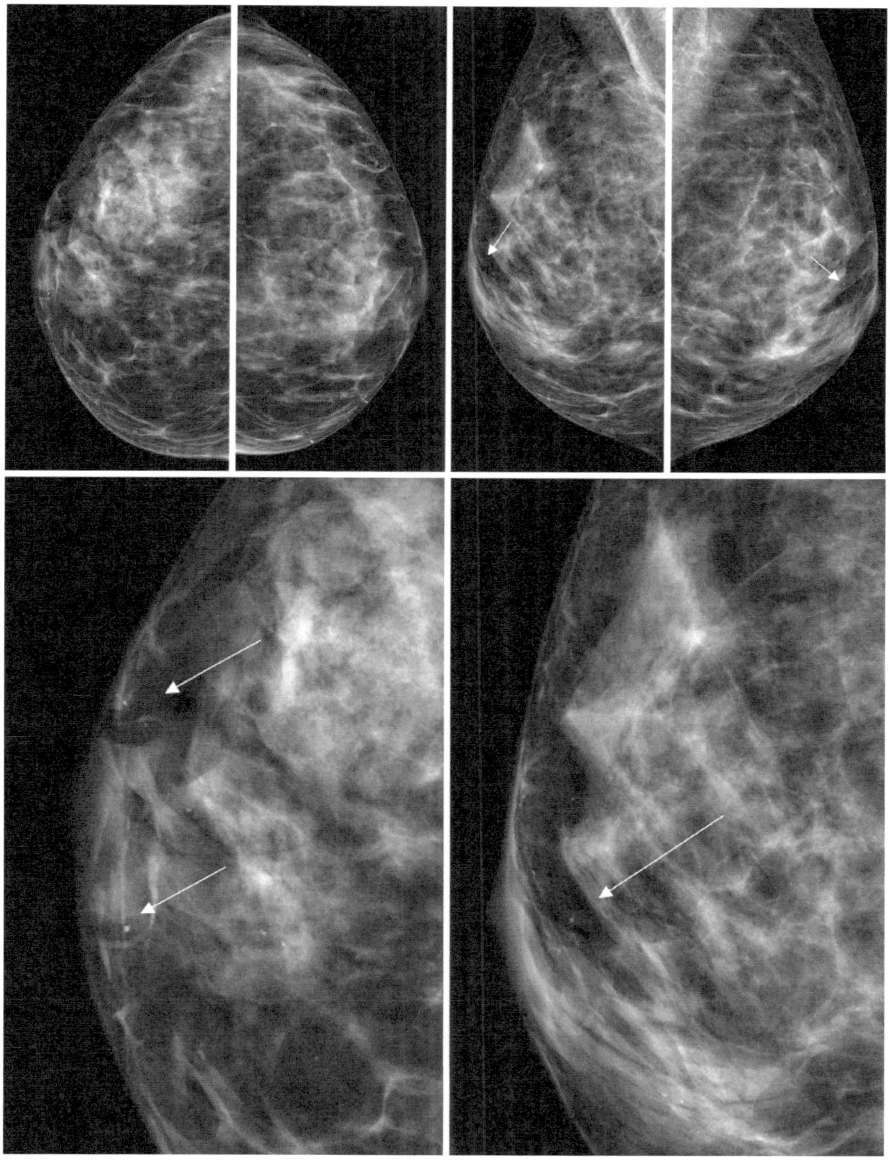

Fig. 3.6 Bilateral mammography and zoomed views retroareolar right. Breast reduction. Breasts of density type c. The gland remodelings related to the mastopexy are barely visible but we note fine round retroareolar microcalcifications of vertical distribution (arrows) and cutaneous, representing the scar path

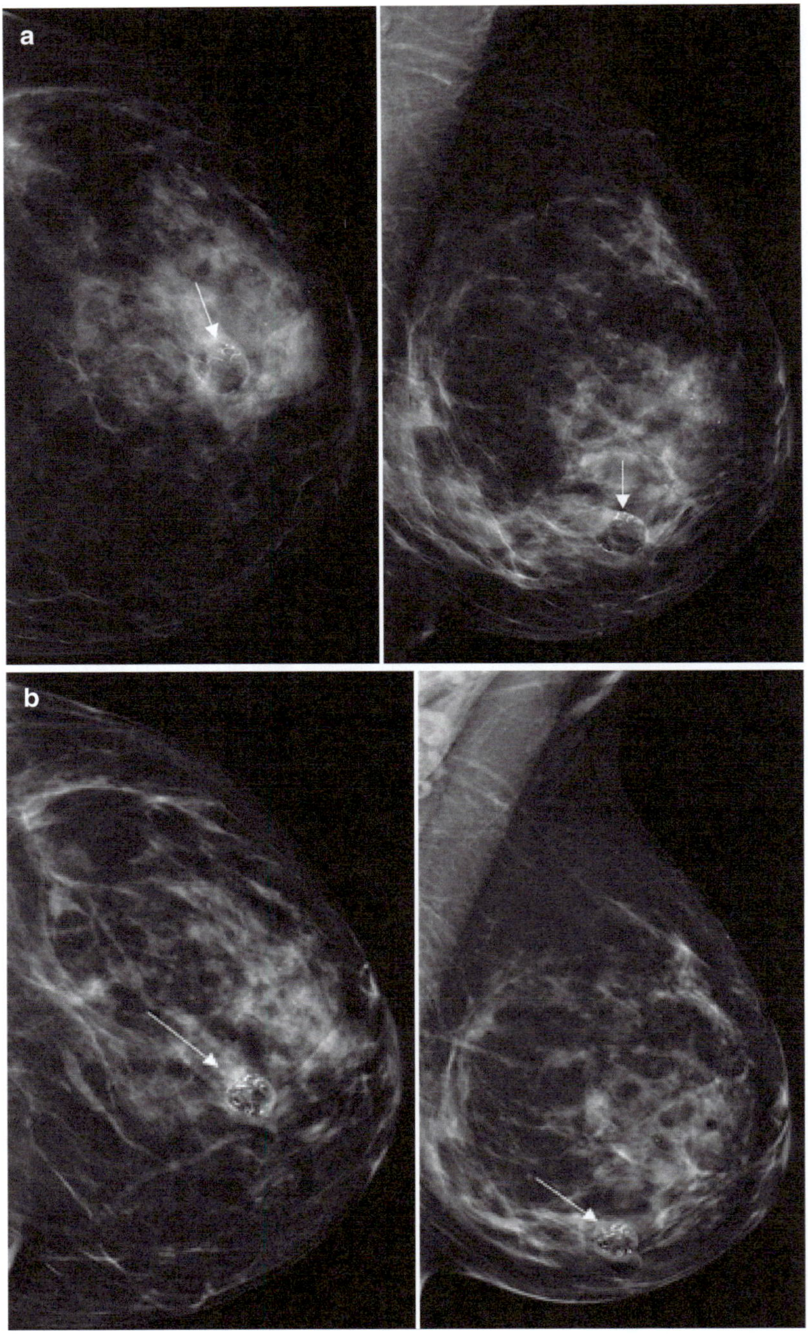

Fig. 3.7 CC and MLO left mammography in the same patient 2 years apart: (**a**) then (**b**). Breast reduction. Fat necrosis. Oil cyst along the mastopexy scar (arrows), of fatty density, with wall calcifications progressing over time

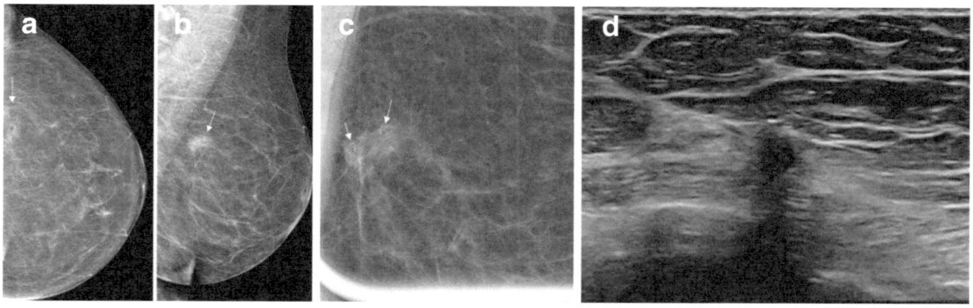

Fig. 3.8 CC and MLO left mammography (**a**, **b**), with magnified lateral view (**c**) and ultrasound (**d**). Breast reduction. Fat necrosis. Misleading appearance. The patient underwent a breast reduction surgery five years ago without any mammography since the procedure. Imaging reveals a centimeter-sized asymmetry accompanied by fine microcalcifications in the upper-outer quadrant of the left breast (**a**, **b**). The additional magnified lateral view performed (**c**), confirms the presence of an asymmetry with oil cysts in contact, presenting eggshell calcifications (arrows). The ultrasound shows a hypoechoic vertically oriented lesion (**d**). A precautionary microbiopsy confirms the presence of fat necrosis

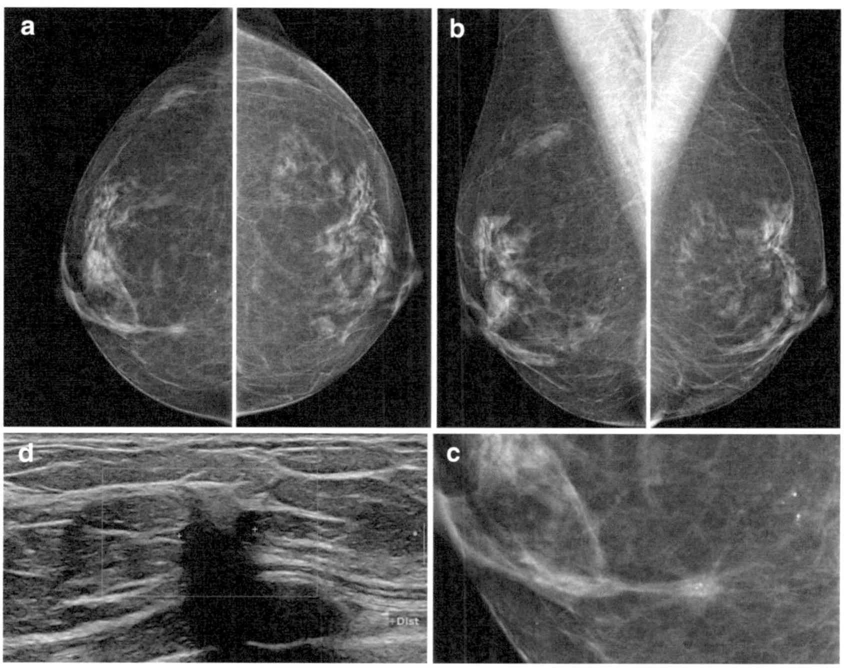

Fig. 3.9 CC and MLO bilateral mammography with zoomed view (**a–c**); Right ultrasound image (**d**). Breast MRI, T1-weighted fat-suppressed MR image in the transverse plane obtained after intravenous administration of a gadolinium chelate (**e**). Fat necrosis. Misleading appearance. The patient underwent a breast reduction three years ago. Clear increase of a spiculated mass, at the junction of the right internal quadrants, with fine microcalcifications (zoomed view). The ultrasound finds a hypoechoic mass with blurry contours, strongly attenuating, suspicious (**d**). The MRI confirms the presence of a spiculated mass showing strong contrast enhancement (**e**). A microbiopsy was performed and revealed Fat necrosis

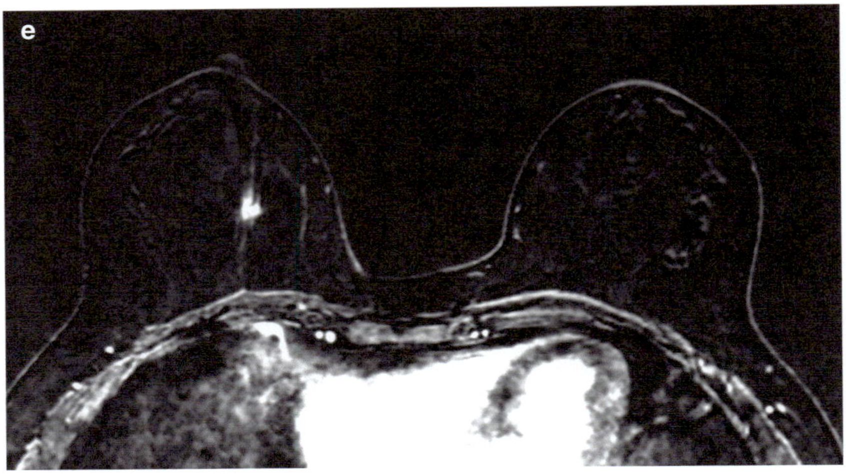

Fig. 3.9 (continued)

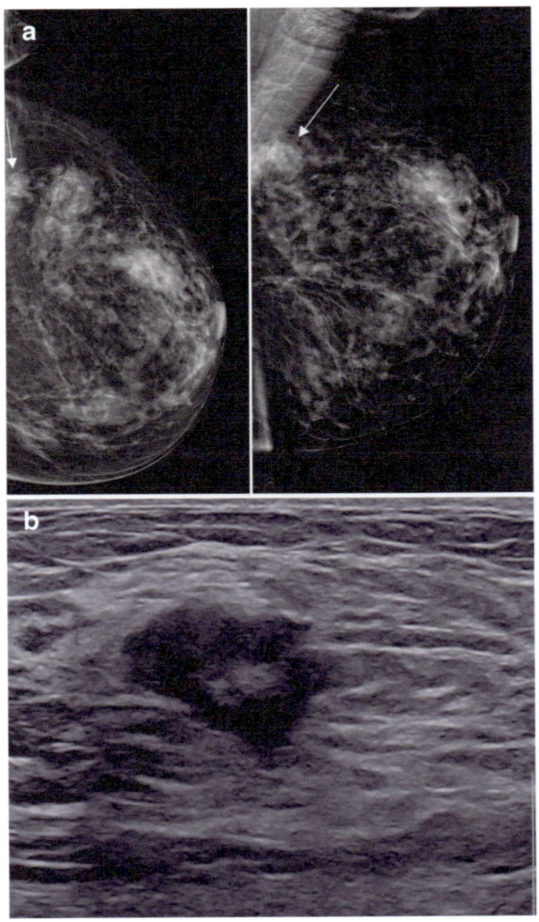

Fig. 3.10 Left CC and MLO mammography and ultrasound. Breast reduction. Appearance of a deep mass with irregular contours of the upper-outer quadrant (**a**) (arrows), corresponding to a hypoechoic lesion, with irregular contours on ultrasound (**b**). Biopsy revealed an invasive ductal carcinoma of intermediate grade. The post-surgical changes do not hinder interpretation because of low breast density in the deeper breast

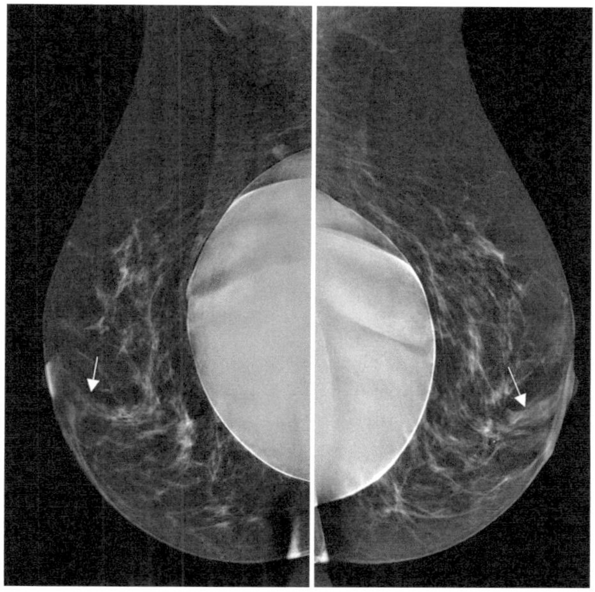

Fig. 3.11 Bilateral mammography in MLO view. Mastopexy to correct ptosis, combined with the placement of retropectoral implants to address insufficient volume. There are thin retroareolar scar bands, concave upwards, witnesses of the mastopexy (arrows). The implant is intact

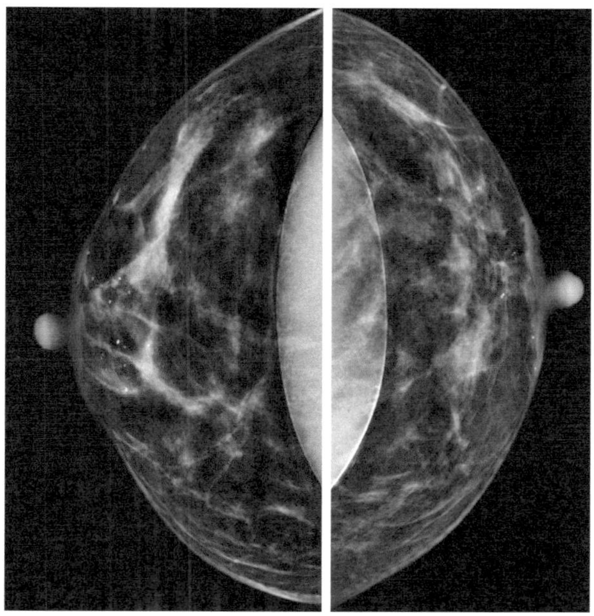

Fig. 3.12 Mammography after mastopexy and placement of implants. No fibrous bands are highlighted but the retroareolar microcalcifications testify to the mastopexy, in addition to the placement of the implants

3.3.2 Ultrasound

Ultrasound becomes increasingly valuable as breast density often rises following a mastopexy or breast reduction. The initial ultrasound conducted post-operatively acts as a baseline for future comparisons.

The ultrasound-guided microbiopsy, can be performed exactly in the same way as without a history of mastopexy.

US may show:

- Areas of attenuation are observed, likely due to scarring, which can variably impact interpretive clarity. These areas typically present as slender, vertical, and linear structures in the orthogonal plane. Notably, the connection of these scars to the skin surface is often discernible, aiding in their identification and assessment during the ultrasound examination (Fig. 3.13).
- Oil cysts: At an early stage, the oil cyst mimics a liquid cyst. At an intermediate stage, the cyst combines an anechoic component and often nodular echoic elements attached to the wall. At a later stage, the appearance is more like a cyst with thick content with attenuating zones related to parietal calcifications [11] (Fig. 3.14). There is never any vascularization of the cyst on doppler.

Ultrasound Appearance

- Attenuating area corresponding to the scars.
- Oil cysts.

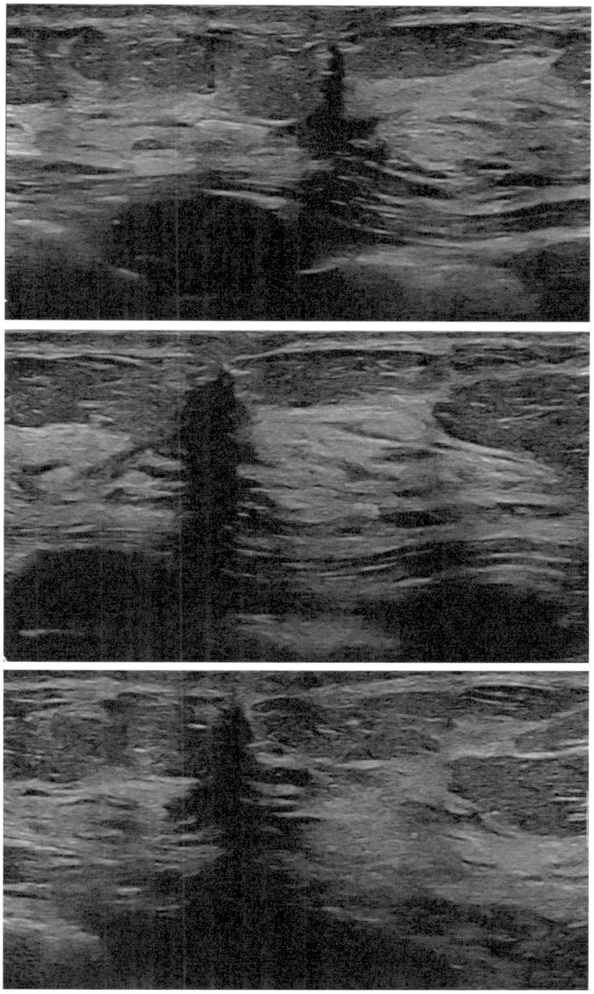

Fig. 3.13 Breast ultrasound (3 successive images at the junction of the lower quadrants). Mastopexy scar. Linear attenuating area changing depending on the positioning of the probe, corresponding to the mastopexy scar. These images are sometimes misleading

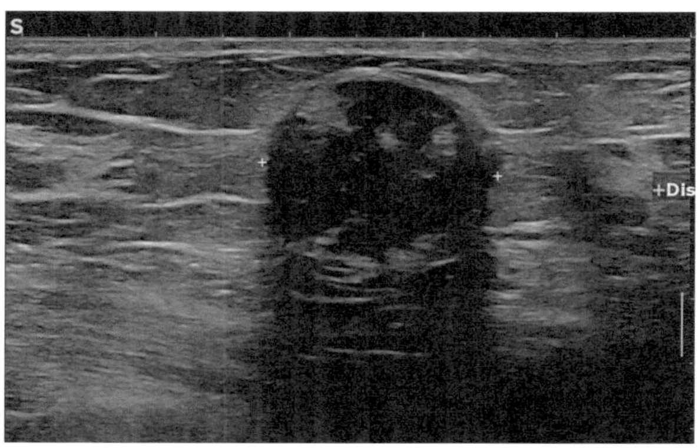

Fig. 3.14 Breast ultrasound. Oil cyst. Typical heterogeneous anechoic round mass with isoechoic portions and attenuating walls, along the mastopexy scar

3.3.3 MRI

MRI is not routinely conducted either before or after breast reduction surgery. However, it becomes pertinent postoperatively if the surgical specimen unexpectedly reveals a lesion. In such cases, the aim is to identify any residual areas of contrast enhancement or to detect lesions in other locations (Fig. 3.15). MRI is also valuable in distinguishing between normal postoperative architectural changes and pathological architectural distortions. There are no specific sequences required beyond the standard breast MRI protocol for these evaluations.

MRI findings:

- Presence of slender fibrous bands exhibiting low signal on both T1 and T2 sequences, without contrast enhancement. These bands are predominantly located in the retroareolar region and lower breast quadrants, and do not impede interpretative accuracy (Figs. 3.16 and 3.17).
- Notable architectural changes of the mammary gland, which are more distinctly observed in the sagittal plane.
- Fat necrosis lesions: The oil cyst, due to its fatty component, takes a characteristic MRI appearance with a hypersignal in T1 and T2 and an absence of signal in case of fat signal saturation. Classically, the oil cyst does not enhance after contrast injection. However, there may be a linear and regular peripheral enhancement due to the attraction of normal vessels, and a scar component associated with it (Fig. 3.17). Sometimes, the oil cyst may appear inflammatory, exhibiting more pronounced contrast uptake that can even seem suspicious [11] (Figs. 3.9 and 3.17).

MRI Appearances

- Fibrous bands.
- Architectural changes.
- Fat necrosis lesions.

It is essential for radiologists to possess a thorough understanding of surgical techniques and the typical postoperative appearances following a breast reduction or mastopexy. This knowledge is crucial in accurately interpreting imaging findings and distinguishing normal post-surgical changes from potential abnormalities. Moreover, imaging of a breast that has undergone reconstruction demands even greater technical precision compared to a non-operated breast. Such rigor ensures accurate assessments, aiding in the early detection of any complications or malignancies, and contributes significantly to the optimal management and follow-up care of these patients.

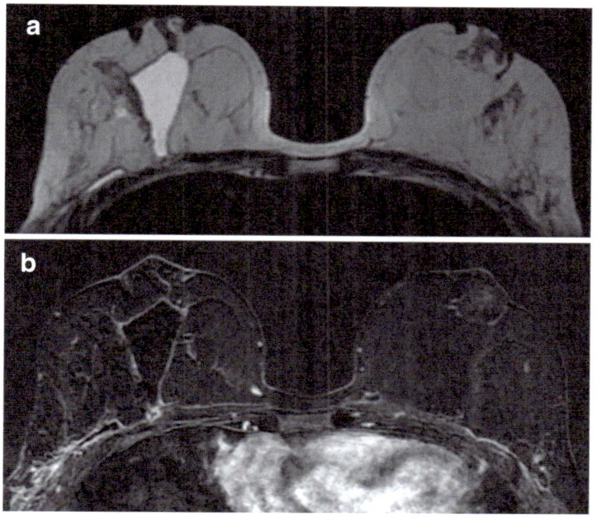

Fig. 3.15 Immediate postoperative breast MRI, conducted following a breast reduction, utilizing sequences T2-weighted (**a**) and T1-weighted fat-suppressed after intravenous administration of a gadolinium chelate (**b**). This MRI was obtained after the discovery of a 3-mm ductal carcinoma in situ on the operative specimen of the left breast, to investigate the presence of any larger, contiguous lesion (the mammography and US had been negative). The imaging revealed a postoperative fluid collection in the right breast, characterized by a bright T2 hypersignal and subtle peripheral contrast enhancement. No suspicious areas of contrast uptake were observed in either breast

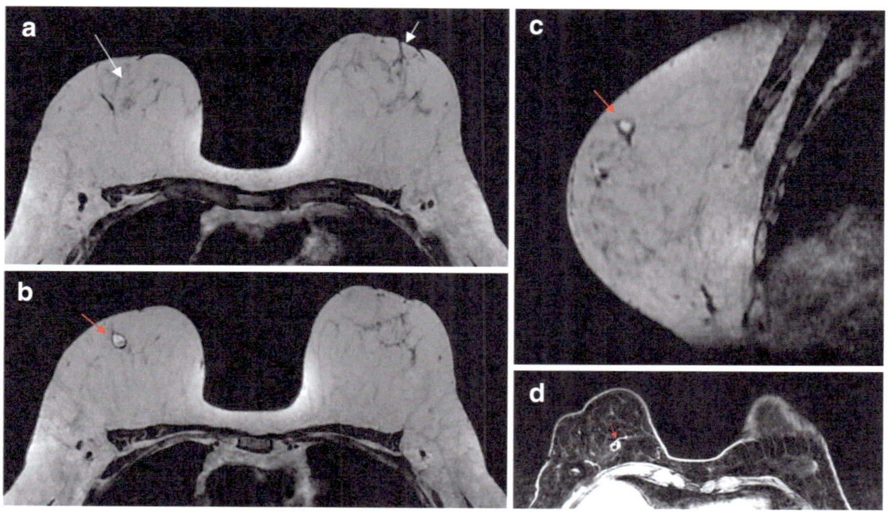

Fig. 3.16 Post-Mastopexy Breast MRI. Axial T1-weighted slices (**a**, **b**), sagittal T1-weighted slice (**c**), and axial T1 fat-suppressed slice 2 min post-contrast injection (**d**). The images reveal extremely fine, bilateral retroareolar scar bands (white arrows). Additionally, small oil cysts in the right breast are visible, displaying high signal intensity on T1 and peripheral enhancement (red arrows)

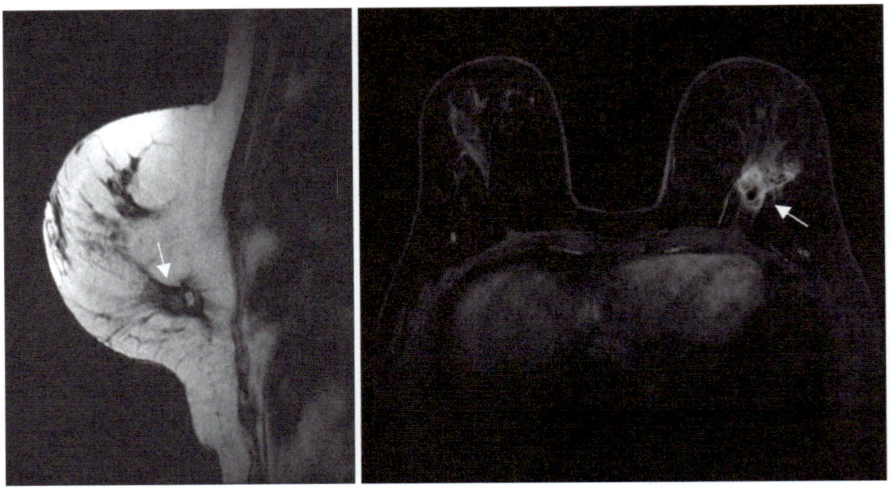

Fig. 3.17 Breast MRI. Sagittal T1 slice of the left breast without fat signal suppression and axial T1-weighted FS post-contrast injection. Fat necrosis. Retroareolar fibrous band with oil cyst in T1 hypersignal at the junction of the lower quadrants of the left breast. After injection and fat signal saturation, there is a thick and irregular inflammatory wall, with a suspicious enhancement pattern. Subsequent biopsy and histological examination reveal inflammatory changes, and no malignant cells were detected

References

1. Yao A, et al. Do larger reductions yield larger returns? Patient-reported outcomes as a function of specimen weight in bilateral reduction mammoplasty. J Plast Reconstr Aesthet Surg. 2021;74:2537.
2. Li Z, et al. Vertical scar versus inverted-T scar reduction Mammaplasty: a meta-analysis and systematic review. Aesth Plast Surg. 2021;45:1385.
3. Pinel-Giroux FM, et al. Breast reconstruction: review of surgical methods and spectrum of imaging findings. Radiographics. 2013;33(2):435–53.
4. Colohan SM, Massenburg BB, Gougoutas AJ. Breast reduction: surgical techniques with an emphasis on evidence-based practice and outcomes. Plast Reconstr Surg. 2020;146(3):339e–50e.
5. Sears ED, et al. Use of preoperative mammography during evaluation for nononcologic breast reduction surgery. JAMA Surg. 2019;154(4):356–8.
6. Klement KA, et al. Discussion of preoperative mammography in women undergoing reduction mammaplasty. Breast J. 2019;25(3):439–43.
7. Broer PN, et al. How to approach secondary breast reduction: international trends and a systematic review of the literature. Aesth Plast Surg. 2021;45:2555.
8. Lowes S, et al. Breast imaging for aesthetic surgery: British Society of Breast Radiology (BSBR), Association of Breast Surgery Great Britain & Ireland (ABS), British Association of Plastic Reconstructive and Aesthetic Surgeons. J Plast Reconstr Aesthet Surg. 2018;71(11):1521.
9. Scaranelo AM, et al. Imaging approaches and findings in the reconstructed breast: a pictorial essay. Can Assoc Radiol J. 2011;62(1):60–72.
10. Roberts JM, et al. Incidence of abnormal mammograms after reduction mammoplasty: implications for oncoplastic closure. Am J Surg. 2011;201(5):611–4.
11. Taboada J, et al. The many faces of fat necrosis in the breast. AJR Am J Roentgenol. 2009;192(3):815–25.

4 Breast Augmentation by Lipofilling

Contents

4.1 Surgical Technique

4.1.1 General Concept

Lipofilling developed thanks to the advent of liposuction in the 1970s, followed by the development of fat reinjection in the 1990s. It involves removing fat from the belly, buttocks, or hips (depending on the patient's morphology) and reinjecting it into the breast to:

- Increase the overall volume of the breast.
- Correct an asymmetry or malformation.
- Fill a defect (post-tumorectomy).
- Complete the reconstruction by implant or flap after mastectomy.

S. Cohen-Zarade, *Imaging of Plastic Surgery of the Breast and Other Implants*,
https://doi.org/10.1007/978-3-031-64159-6_4

Lipofilling is a rapidly expanding technique, very popular with patients, for several reasons:

- There is no visible scar: the fat is introduced through micro-incisions of 1 mm.
- There is no foreign body, so there is no implant monitoring or reoperation to plan for their renewal.

4.1.2 Procedure

It is an autograft of adipocytes. No foreign body is implanted in the body [1].

The fat is removed then centrifuged to be purified and to extract the intact adipocytes. It is then delicately reinjected into the breast.

The procedure is performed under general anesthesia and often in several sessions (Fig. 4.1).

Lipofilling can be combined with the placement of breast implants or be performed after removal of implants, in addition to a mastopexy, to restore volume.

4.1.3 Risk of Carcinogenesis

There was initially controversy among patients treated for breast cancer, with flap or implant reconstruction, supplemented by lipofilling. Indeed, given the possible fat-breast gland interactions, a hypothetical risk of stimulating carcinogenesis due to the richness of fat in stem cells and the presence of growth factors in the centrifugation fluid was discussed, but various studies have not corroborated this hypothesis [2].

To fill defects after conservative treatment, a delay of 2 years is often respected before performing lipofilling.

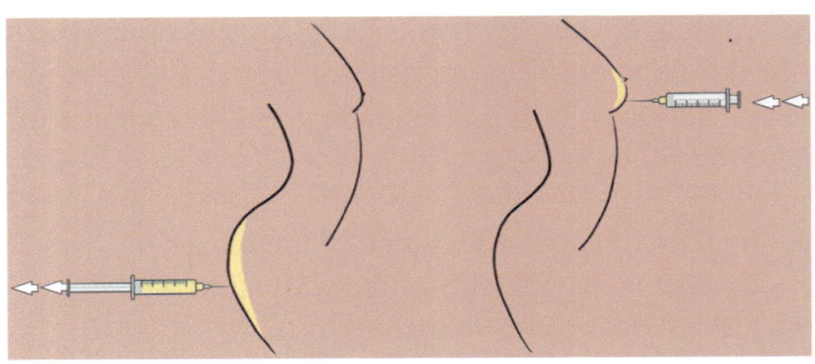

Fig. 4.1 Lipofilling diagram. Removal of buttock fat and intramammary reinjection after centrifugation. (*Drawing by Jean-Charles Goldberg*)

4.2 Imaging Protocol

- **The standard pre-operative assessment** includes a mammogram with two 2D views (CC and MLO), a tomosynthesis acquisition, and an ultrasound depending on the breast density [3].

Any lesion classified as ACR4, ACR5 or even ACR3 must be biopsied for histological analysis, before surgery [1, 4].

There is no formal consensus to date, but most surgeons prefer the mammography to be 6 months to 1 year before the procedure.

The age of realization is mandatory after 40 years. In patients between the ages of 30 and 40, the pre-surgical evaluation typically includes an ultrasound and sometimes a single mediolateral oblique (MLO) mammogram view of each breast, looking for microcalcifications.

MRI is often performed preoperatively as a reference assessment and is always recommended for patients with a history of breast cancer [5, 6].

- **Postoperative imaging** is not systematically performed because immediate postoperative complications are rare, if not exceptional (infectious mastitis).
- **The follow-up** is identical to that of the general population. Lipofilling does not increase the risk of developing a breast cancer.

4.3 Imaging Appearances

The aspects are typical but can be misleading if they are unknown [7, 8]. They do not interfere with the detection of breast cancer during follow-up and do not alter the diagnostic performance of imaging examinations.

4.3.1 Mammography

- In 75% of cases, we can see small **oil cysts** less than 1 cm in size with calcified or non-calcified walls, which are not a complication of the procedure, but the normal appearance after lipofilling (Figs. 4.2 and 4.3).
- Some oil cysts can become inflammatory, increasing in size, with wall thickening and calcifications, forming a **fat necrosis** (Fig. 4.2). These can be palpable and be a reason for the patient's consultation, who must then be reassured. The risk of developing them increases with the amount of fat injected [6].

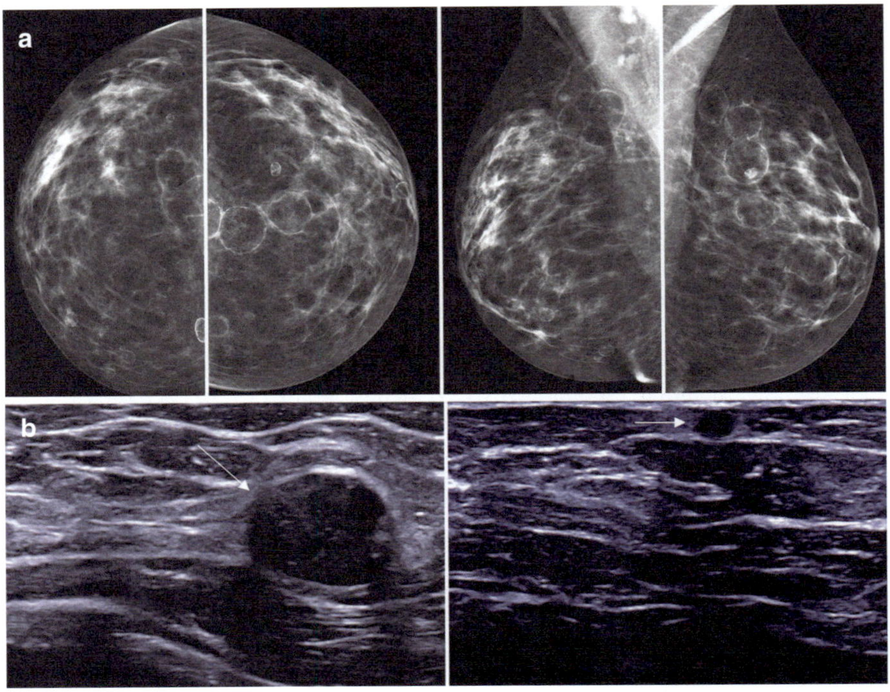

Fig. 4.2 Bilateral mammography and two breast ultrasound images. Lipofilling. (**a**) The mammogram shows oil cysts of different sizes on both sides. Some have a calcified wall. (**b**) The ultrasound finds lesions of fat necrosis and superficial oil microcysts

- An increase in the thickness of the retroglandular fat may be observed when comparing post-operative mammograms to those taken prior to the intervention (Fig. 4.4).
- Calcifications with a benign appearance may emerge, often scattered throughout the tissue (Fig. 4.4).

Lipofilling on Mammography

- Oil cysts.
- Increase in the thickness of the retroglandular fat.
- Calcifications.

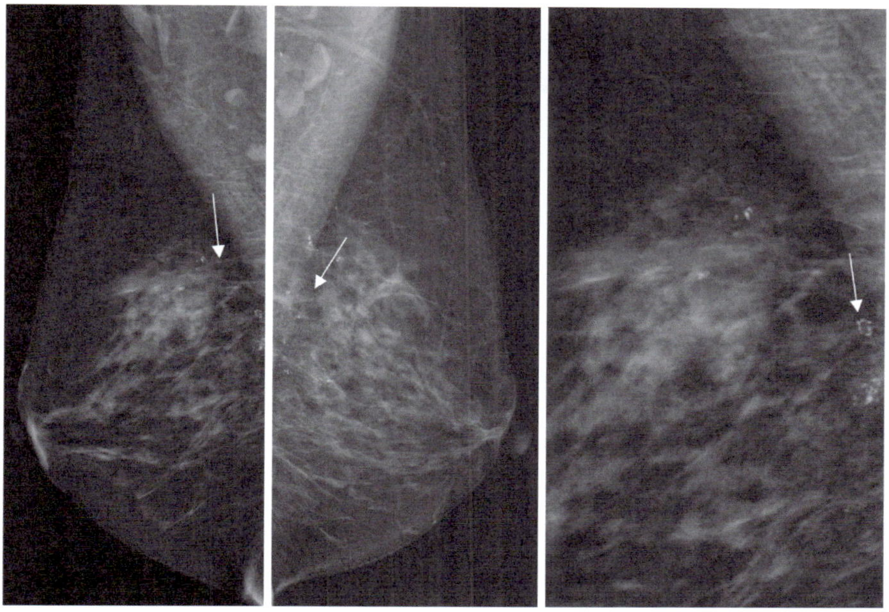

Fig. 4.3 Bilateral mammography in MLO view and zoomed view. Lipofilling. We visualize some deep calcified oil microcysts, better visible on the zoomed view. Obtaining a good patient history is essential because the aspect is less suggestive than in the previous figure

When encountering imaging findings indicative of lipofilling, it is crucial to directly inquire with the patient regarding their surgical history. Patients may not always voluntarily disclose having undergone such procedures, making proactive questioning by the healthcare provider essential for accurate medical evaluation and diagnosis (Fig. 4.3).

In the specific case of lipofilling performed after explantation of implants associated with a mastopexy, we visualize both the stigmata of lipofilling and those of the mastopexy (Fig. 4.5).

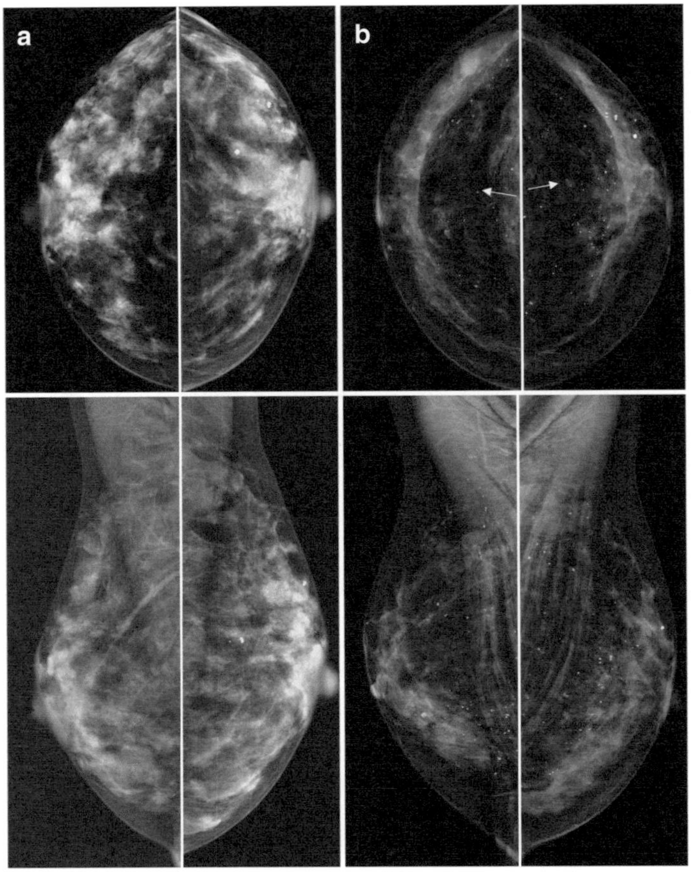

Fig. 4.4 CC and MLO mammography before (**a**) and after (**b**) lipofilling. After lipofilling (**b**), there is a large thickness of the retroglandular fat (white arrows) compared to the preoperative mammogram (**a**), due to the good effectiveness of the autograft. In addition, appearance of dense, non-suspicious bilateral scattered microcalcifications

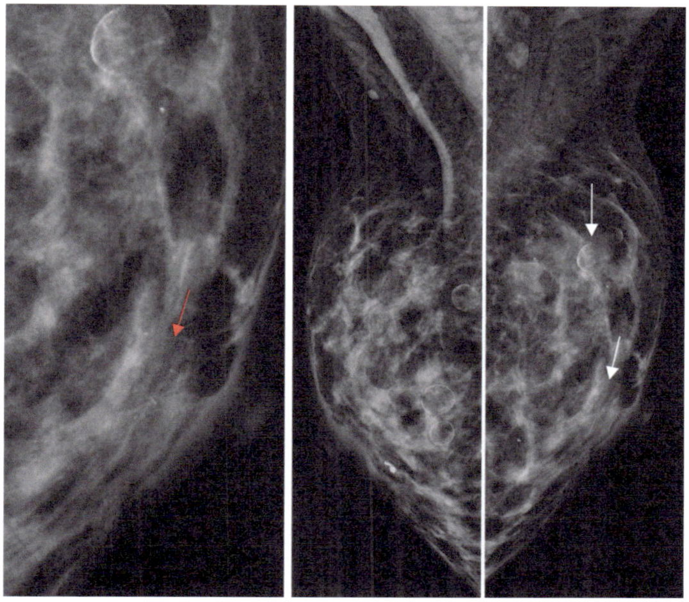

Fig. 4.5 Bilateral mammography in MLO view and zoomed retroareolar left view. Lipofilling and mastopexy after implant extraction. This patient chose to have her implants removed a few years after they were initially placed. A mastopexy combined with lipofilling allowed to restore volume and drape the skin. There are fine retroareolar microcalcifications related to the mastopexy (red arrow) and oil cysts, some with calcified walls, related to the lipofilling (white arrows)

4.3.2 Ultrasound

- Post-lipofilling, the presence of oil cysts can be observed. These differ from typical cysts by having a thinner wall and being situated within the fatty tissue of the breast rather than the glandular tissue (Figs. 4.2 and 4.6). They are usually small, measuring less than 5 mm in diameter. Such characteristics are considered a normal post-lipofilling manifestation [6].
- Some can be larger and inflammatory.

4.3.3 MRI

In MRI, oil cysts can also be detected. Characteristically, they exhibit high signal intensity in both T1 and T2 sequences without fat suppression and appear as low signal following fat saturation. Additionally, their walls may show subtle contrast enhancement (Figs. 4.6, 4.7 and 4.8).

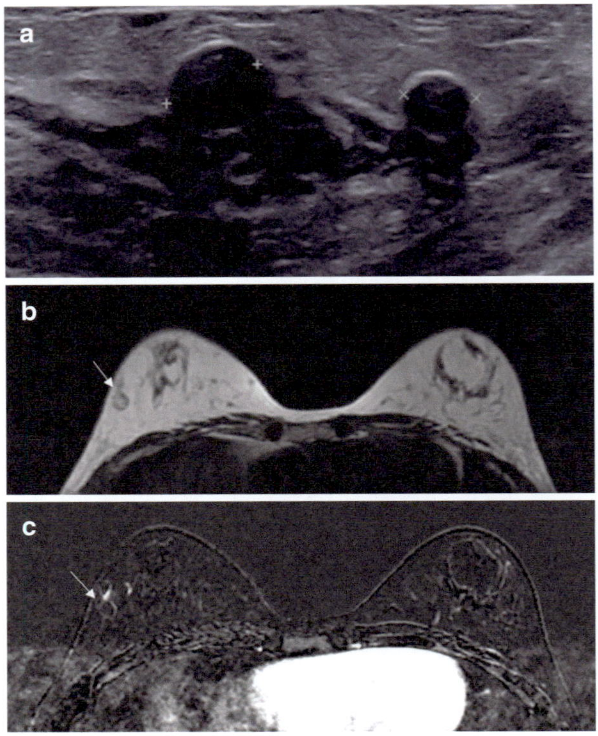

Fig. 4.6 Breast ultrasound (**a**) and breast MRI: T1 sequence without fat signal saturation (**b**) and T1-weighted imaging post-contrast with fat suppression (**c**). Lipofilling. (**a**) Oil cysts with very finely calcified walls. (**b**) Typical lipofilling image in the form of an oil cyst with a thin wall, hyperintense on T1W sequence. (**c**) Very subtle enhancement of the cyst wall, not significant and not suspicious

An inflammatory appearance with significant contrast uptake should lead to a biopsy to differentiate an inflammatory fat necrosis from a progressive lesion (Fig. 4.9).

Lipofilling, offering augmentation without the introduction of foreign bodies, presents unique advantages over traditional breast implants. It's crucial for radiologists specializing in breast imaging to have a comprehensive understanding of the typical imaging features associated with fat grafting, as well as its potential complications. This knowledge is key for accurate diagnosis and management, as the imaging manifestations of lipofilling can differ significantly from those associated with implants. Recognizing both normal post-lipofilling appearances and signs of complications ensures high-quality patient care and informed clinical decision-making in the field of breast imaging.

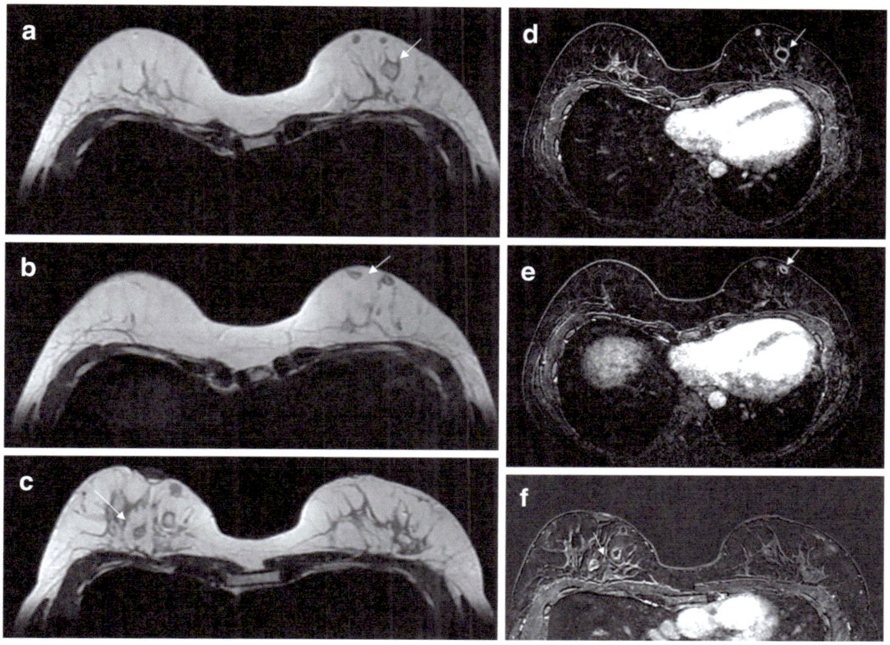

Fig. 4.7 Breast MRI. Lipofilling: (**a**–**c**) T1 sequence without fat signal saturation: Typical lipofilling images in the form of small oil cysts with thin walls, hyperintense on T1W sequence. (**d**–**f**) T1-weighted imaging post-contrast with fat suppression: Very fine contrast uptake of the cyst wall, not significant and not suspicious

Fig. 4.8 Breast MRI. (**a**) T1 sequence without fat signal saturation. A dominant hyperintense oil cyst on the right in T1W imaging, featuring calcified areas appearing as signal voids. Adjacent are smaller cysts with similar characteristics. (**b**) T1-weighted imaging post-contrast with fat suppression. Lipofilling. Fine contrast uptake of the oil cyst wall, not suspicious

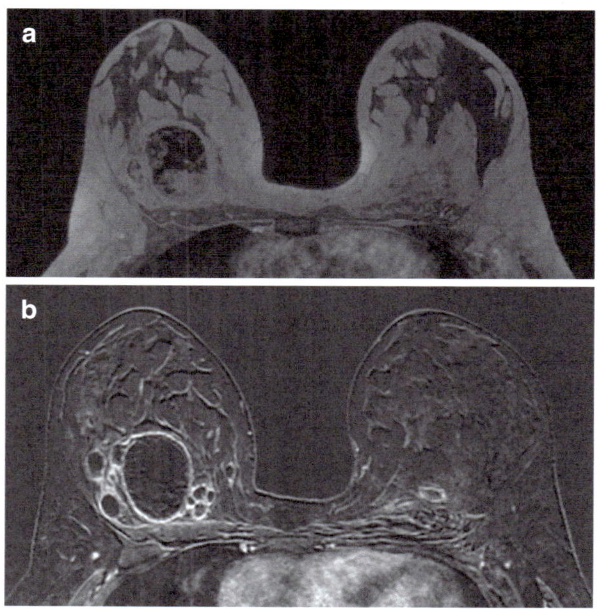

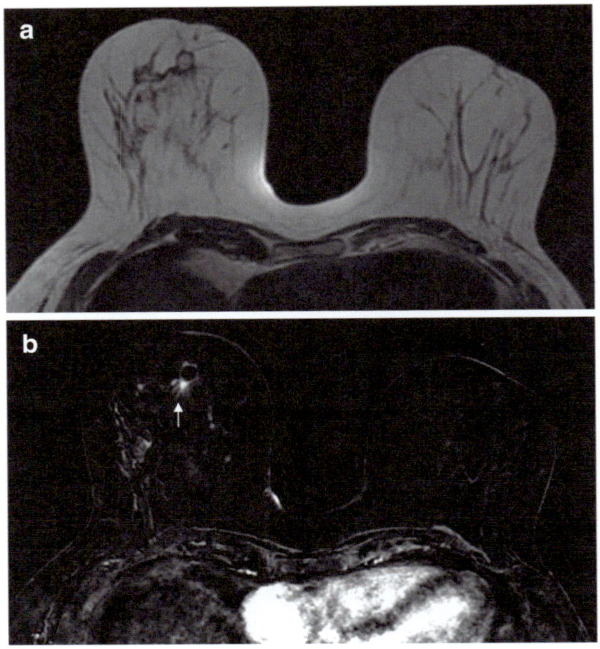

Fig. 4.9 Breast MRI T1 sequence without fat signal saturation (**a**) and T1 2 minu after injection and fat signal saturation (**b**). Lipofilling Right retroareolar oil cyst appearing hyperintense in T1W and hypointense after injection and fat signal saturation. There is a thick and pseudo-spiculated posterior wall contrast uptake that led to an ultrasound-guided microbiopsy. Histology confirmed the existence of a simple fat necrosis without associated malignancy

References

1. Hanson SE, Kapur SK. Oncologic safety and surveillance of autologous fat grafting following breast conservation therapy. Plast Reconstr Surg. 2020;146(2):215–25.
2. Krastev T, Jonasse Y, Kon K. Oncological safety of autologous lipoaspirate grafting in breast cancer patients: a systematic review. Ann Surg Oncol. 2013;20(1):111–9.
3. Carloni R, et al. Preoperative imaging prior to breast reconstruction surgery: benchmarking bringing together radiologists and plastic surgeons. Proposed guidelines. Ann Chir Plast Esthet. 2014;59(2):e13–9.
4. Rubin JP, et al. Mammographic changes after fat transfer to the breast compared with changes after breast reduction: a blinded study. Plast Reconstr Surg. 2012;129(5):1029–38.
5. Margolis NE, et al. Update on imaging of the postsurgical breast. Radiographics. 2014;34(3):642–60.
6. Pinell-White XA, et al. Radiographic implications of fat grafting to the reconstructed breast. Breast J. 2015;21(5):520–5.
7. Costantini M, et al. Radiological findings in mammary autologous fat injections: a multi-technique evaluation. Clin Radiol. 2013;68(1):27–33.
8. Lindegren A, et al. Autologous fat transplantation to the reconstructed breast does not hinder assessment of mammography and ultrasound: a cohort study. World J Surg. 2016;40(5):1104–11.

Less Conventional Breast Augmentation Techniques

5

Contents

Alternative aesthetic procedures, which are less commonly performed or even prohibited, still require awareness by medical professionals. Understanding both the normal and pathological manifestations of these procedures is crucial for accurate interpretation of diagnostic imaging. This knowledge guides the radiologist in determining the appropriate imaging assessment and ensures comprehensive evaluation, especially in cases where patients may not voluntarily disclose their surgical history. Such expertise is key in identifying potential complications arising from these less conventional methods.

5.1 Intramammary Free Silicone Injection

5.1.1 Surgical Technique

Free silicone injection can be practiced anywhere in the body. Large volumes are injected into the breasts, buttocks, or calves [1]. Unlike hyaluronic acid, which is biocompatible and degradable, silicone remains a permanent filler product that

S. Cohen-Zarade, *Imaging of Plastic Surgery of the Breast and Other Implants*,
https://doi.org/10.1007/978-3-031-64159-6_5

cannot be completely eliminated by the body. Its use was widespread in the 1960s and then banned in the 90 s. Tolerance is often poor in the long term, with the appearance of pain and granulomas.

5.1.2 Imaging Protocol

The follow-up assessment includes:

- A standard mammogram with 2 2D views and a tomosynthesis.
- An ultrasound.
- An MRI.

5.1.3 Imaging Appearances

Mammography

The interpretive accuracy of the mammography is significantly compromised by the presence of densely coalesced masses within the breast parenchyma. These masses are identified as siliconomas, and their presence can obscure and complicate the evaluation of the underlying breast tissue, posing challenges in distinguishing between normal structures and potential pathologies [2] (Figs. 5.1 and 5.2).

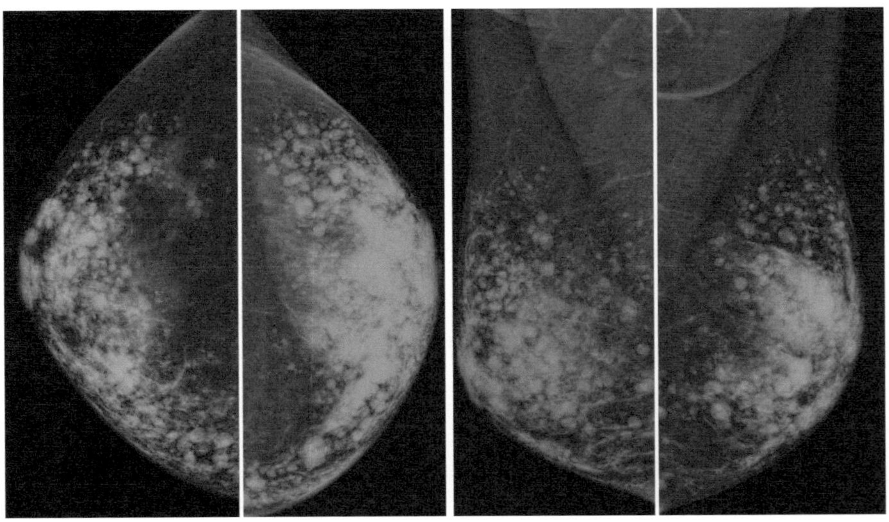

Fig. 5.1 Bilateral mammography. Intra-mammary free silicone injection. Numerous siliconomas, varying in size and density, are present and confluent, severely obstructing the interpretive process of the mammogram. Additionally, the cosmetic outcome was not favorable, characterized by hardened breast tissue and visible "granular" deformations

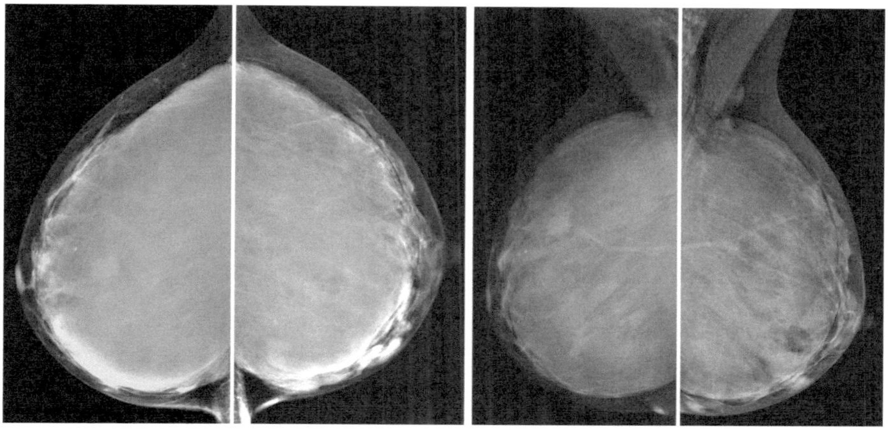

Fig. 5.2 Bilateral mammography. Intra-mammary free silicone injection

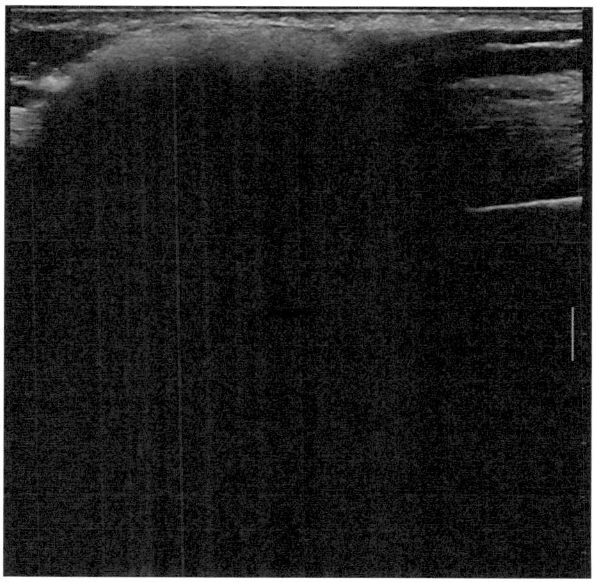

Fig. 5.3 Breast ultrasound. Intramammary free silicone injection. Large attenuating siliconoma with a "snowstorm" appearance that hinders interpretation

Each breast features a dominant siliconoma, accompanied by several smaller siliconomas. These could be mistaken for breast implants due to their size and placement, if not for their distinct density and less defined borders. The aesthetic result was satisfactory.

Ultrasound

The masses appear as attenuating pseudo-cysts with varying degrees of coalescence and are dispersed throughout the breast tissue, giving a “snowstorm” appearance. This term describes how the non-encapsulated silicone irregularly distributes itself within the breast tissue. The pseudo-cysts represent accumulations of silicone, varying in size and shape (Fig. 5.3).

MRI

This examination is the most suitable for analyzing the distribution of the substance and visualizing more obscured breast tissue. The MRI protocol, in addition to standard sequences, necessitates:

- T2 sequences with **fat saturation**: the liquid and hyaluronic acid appear in high signal.
- WATER STIR "**silicone only**" sequences: The silicone appears in high signal.

This allows us to differentiate the different injected components (Fig. 5.4).

These sequences are typically performed in two different planes, axial and sagittal, to provide a comprehensive view of the breast. The axial plane is valuable for evaluating the overall distribution and extent of the silicone, while the sagittal plane offers a detailed view of the anterior-posterior aspect. This multiplanar approach ensures a thorough assessment, helping to map out the exact locations and volumes of the silicone injections.

Same patient as in Fig. 5.2. The observations are like those in the mammography, with a primary siliconoma in each breast and additional confluent siliconomas in proximity. Diagnosing potential breast cancer is extremely challenging due to this widespread masking effect. However, the cosmetic outcome was satisfactory.

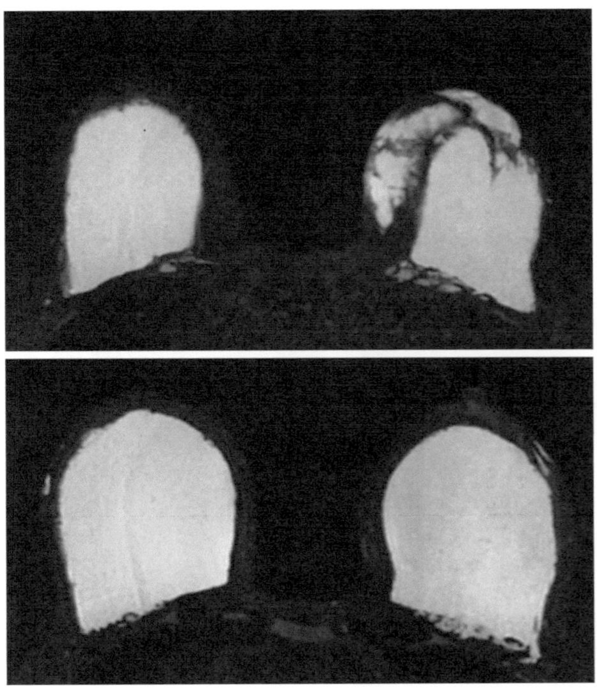

Fig. 5.4 Breast MRI. Intramammary free silicone injection. "Silicone only" sequence

5.2 Intramammary Free Hyaluronic Acid Injection

5.2.1 Surgical Technique

This intervention is still performed in some countries, even if it is not recommended.

Hyaluronic acid has a volumizing power due to the attraction of water molecules [3, 4].

The market offers a wide range of hyaluronic acid products. For breast augmentation, a denser variant of hyaluronic acid is used compared to that for treating facial wrinkles. The selection of a particular product depends on various factors, such as viscosity and the degree of cross-linking, tailored to the desired outcome and longevity of the effect [5]. The effects of hyaluronic acid as a filler are temporary, as the body gradually metabolizes it. The duration of visible effects and the rate at which the body absorbs the filler can vary, making this a significant consideration in patient counseling [6, 7].

5.2.2 Imaging Protocol

The follow-up assessment includes:

- A standard mammography with 2 2D views and a tomosynthesis.
- An ultrasound.
- An MRI.

Imaging Appearances

Mammography

Hyaluronic acid injections create confluent, scattered, and relatively dense masses within the breast tissue. These masses typically appear less dense than silicone, which is an important distinction in mammographic interpretation, particularly in breast cancer screening (Figs. 5.5a and 5.6a).

Ultrasound

The imaging reveals variable-sized pseudocysts. The absence of a “snowstorm” appearance, which is characteristic of siliconoma, is a key differentiator. This feature aids clinicians in distinguishing between hyaluronic acid injections and other substances like silicone (Figs. 5.5b and 5.6b–d).

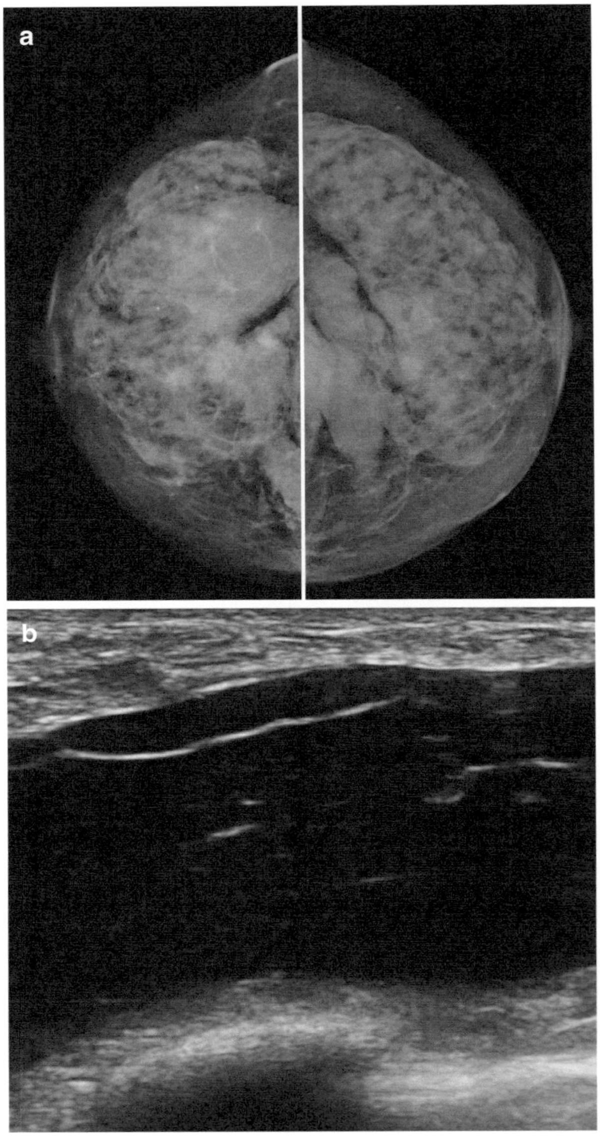

Fig. 5.5 Free hyaluronic acid injection at 6 months. (**a**) Bilateral mammography. The diffusely distributed substance appears less dense than silicone, yet the breast parenchyma remains obscured by dense, confluent clusters. (**b**) Breast ultrasound, image of the right breast. A slightly heterogeneous liquid pseudocyst is formed by the injected product

MRI

It also shows confluent and scattered pseudocysts, in T2 intense high signal, and in low signal on the WATER STIR "silicone only" sequence, in contrast to silicone.

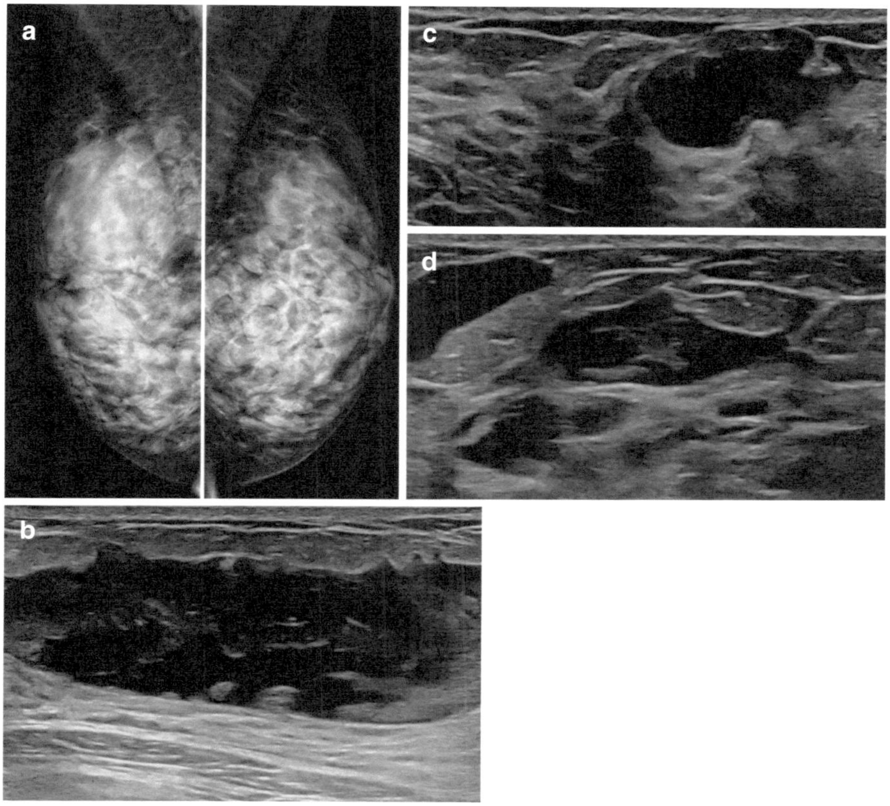

Fig. 5.6 Free hyaluronic acid injection at 4 months. 23-year-old patient who recently had a free hyaluronic acid injection. There are palpable sensitive nodules on clinical examination. (**a**) Bilateral mammography in MLO view. Dense, confluent masses, masking the breast parenchyma. (**b–d**): Three successive images of breast ultrasound. Anechoic pseudocysts with non-vascularized echogenic portions, formed by the product clusters

References

1. Bhardwaj P, et al. Free silicone injections to the breast: delayed complications and surgical management of sequelae. Plast Reconstr Surg Glob Open. 2020;8(11):e3208.
2. Scaranelo A, De Fatima Ribeiro Maia M. Sonographic and mammographic findings of breast liquid silicone injection. J Clin Ultrasound. 2006;34(6):273–7.
3. Fallico N, et al. Augmentation mammaplasty after breast enhancement with macrolane. Plast Reconstr Surg. 2014;133(3):439e–40e.
4. Scaperrotta G, et al. Radiological assessment of the breast following enhancement with macrolane: managing the challenges. Eur J Radiol. 2017;86:58–62.

5. Becchere MP, et al. A case series study on complications after breast augmentation with macrolane. Aesth Plast Surg. 2013;37(2):332–5.
6. Trignano E, et al. Augmentation Mammaplasty after breast enhancement with hyaluronic acid. Aesthet Surg J. 2015;35(6):nP161–8.
7. Trignano E, et al. Complications after breast augmentation with hyaluronic acid: a case report. Gland Surg. 2020;9(6):2193–7.

Male Breast Reduction Surgery

6

Contents

Men can experience an increase in breast size, which may cause aesthetic and social discomfort [1].

This can be due to:

- Gynecomastia: where the increase in volume is primarily glandular. It is the most common cause of breast enlargement in men and represents the majority of cases when men seek consultation for increased breast volume, especially during periods of hormonal changes such as puberty and old age. Gynecomastia can present as:
  - Nodular: It is a form of gynecomastia where the breast tissue enlargement is characterized by a firm, rubbery mass located underneath the nipple area (Fig. 6.1).
  - Dendritic: It is a variant of gynecomastia where the breast tissue, particularly the glandular component, exhibits a branching or tree-like pattern that extends from the nipple area into the surrounding fatty tissue of the chest (Fig. 6.2).
  - Diffuse: It is a form of gynecomastia characterized by a widespread, uniform enlargement of the glandular breast tissue across the breast area, rather than localized nodular or dendritic growth (Fig. 6.3).
- Adipomastia: where the increase in volume is homogeneously fatty. It is strictly related to fat accumulation and does not involve any change in the glandular structure of the breast.There are no distinct masses or nodular densities that might suggest the presence of glandular breast tissue (Fig. 6.4).
- Breast cancer.

S. Cohen-Zarade, *Imaging of Plastic Surgery of the Breast and Other Implants*,
https://doi.org/10.1007/978-3-031-64159-6_6

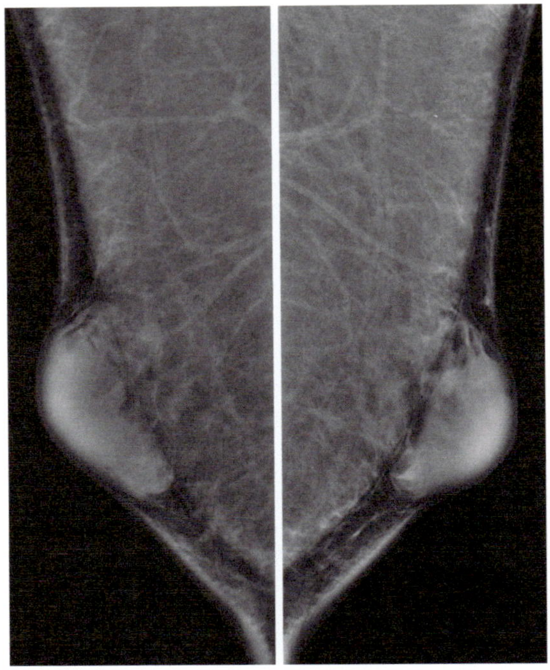

Fig. 6.1 Bilateral mammography in MLO view. Nodular Gynecomastia. The glandular component, well defined, predominates over the fatty component

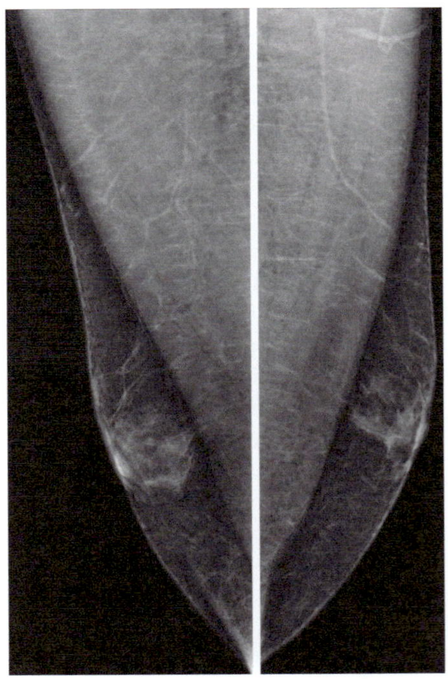

Fig. 6.2 Bilateral mammography in MLO view. Dendritic Gynecomastia. The glandular component, retro-areolar with an indistinct posterior boundary, predominates over the fatty component

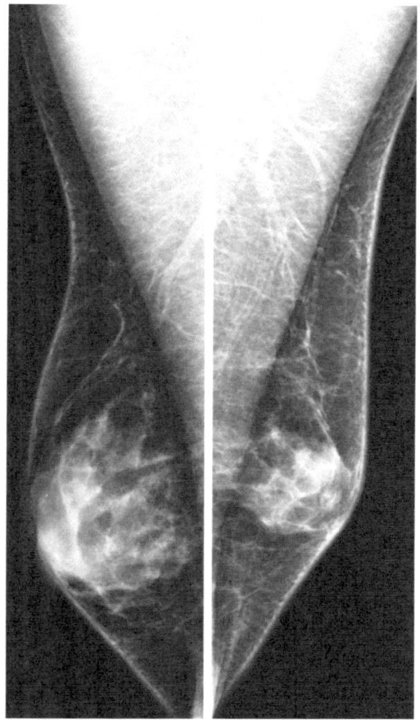

Fig. 6.3 Bilateral mammography in MLO view. Diffuse Gynecomastia. Enlargement of glandular breast tissue characteristic of diffuse gynecomastia, affecting the entire chest area. There is no suspicious mass

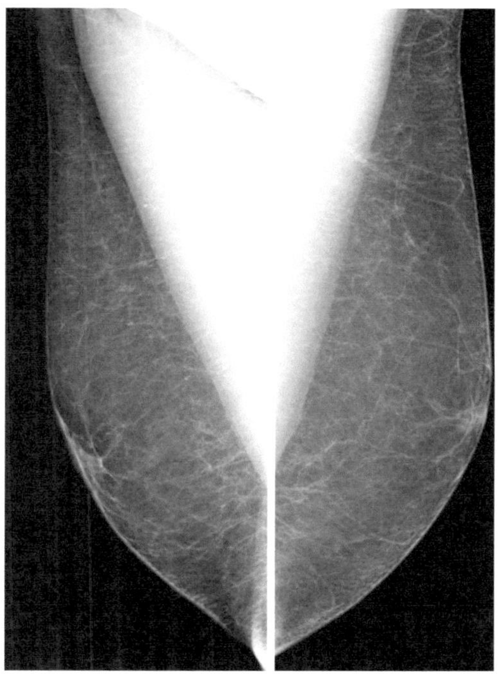

Fig. 6.4 Right and left mammography in MLO view. Adipomastia. The mammogram shows an exclusive adipomastia, characterized by an increased deposition of fatty tissue in the chest region, presenting a radiolucent appearance compared to the denser glandular tissue.It is accessible to liposuction

6.1 Surgical Technique

A preoperative imaging assessment is essential to determine whether to perform a subcutaneous mastectomy for gynecomastia, or liposuction in cases where adipomastia is predominant [2, 3].

6.2 Imaging Protocol

Preoperative procedures include:

- An MLO view mammogram of each breast, comparative, to differentiate the gland from the fat.
- An ultrasound, to look for any additional pathology.

It is not necessary to perform postoperative imaging or follow-up.

6.3 Preoperative Imaging Appearance

The overall gland/fat distribution is more easily interpretable on the mammogram than on the ultrasound. Thus, we distinguish between gynecomastia (Figs. 6.1,6.2 and 6.3) and adipomastia (Fig. 6.4), or the mixed appearance, and we assess the extent and distribution for each breast.

In the case of predominant gynecomastia, we differentiate between nodular gynecomastia (Fig. 6.1), dendritic (Fig. 6.2), diffuse (Fig. 6.3).

Although ultrasound is less effective in assessing the overall distribution of glandular tissue compared to fat, it is valuable for identifying progressive pathologies. This limitation is due to the operator-dependent nature of ultrasound, which tends to provide a more localized perspective rather than a holistic overview (Fig. 6.5).

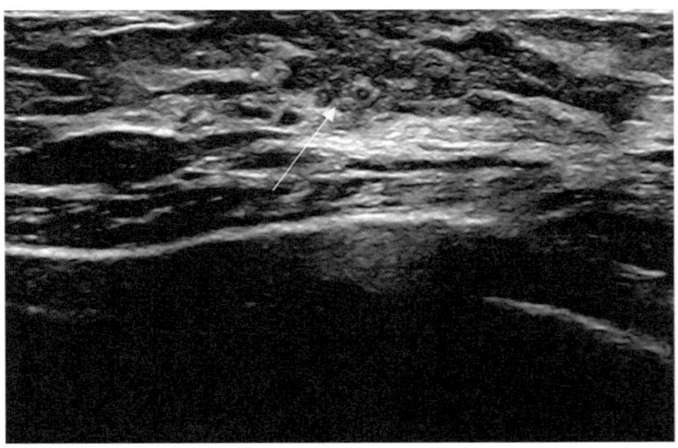

Fig. 6.5 Left breast ultrasound. Gynecomastia. Dendritic retro-areolar gynecomastia in a 25-year-old patient

The imaging plays a crucial role in male breast reduction procedures, primarily for diagnosing conditions like gynecomastia or adipomastia and guiding surgical planning [4]. Imaging techniques like ultrasound and mammography are instrumental in differentiating between glandular and fatty tissue enlargement, thereby determining the most appropriate surgical approach. This comprehensive imaging approach ensures both effective treatment and patient satisfaction.

References

1. Whitehead IJ, et al. Gynaecomastia: a cosmetic concern or a concerning clinical sign? Ann R Coll Surg Engl. 2019;101(8):e184–6.
2. Billa E, Kanakis GA, Goulis DG. Imaging in gynecomastia. Andrology. 2021;9:1444.
3. Yoon B, et al. Male patients with unilateral breast symptoms: an optimal imaging approach. Eur Radiol. 2020;30(8):4242–50.
4. Onder O, et al. Imaging findings and classification of the common and uncommon male breast diseases. Insights Imaging. 2020;11(1):27.

Other Implants

7

Contents

7.1 Buttock and Calf Implants

7.1.1 Surgical Techniques

Buttock Implants

The buttock implant recreates volume and projection to the buttock (Fig. 7.1). The incision is in the inter-buttock fold, at the top of the groove. The intramuscular lodge is made in the thickness of the gluteus maximus muscle, for the placement of the implant [1, 2] (Fig. 7.2). The procedure can be combined with liposuction, a lipofilling or an injection of filler (Figs. 7.3 and 7.4).

Calf Implants

The purpose of calf implants is to enhance the curvature of the calf. The surgical incision is made in the popliteal fossa. The implant is strategically placed between the two heads of the gastrocnemius muscle and within their fascial covering, which helps to conceal its edges and create a natural contour." [3–6] (Fig. 7.5).

S. Cohen-Zarade, *Imaging of Plastic Surgery of the Breast and Other Implants*,
https://doi.org/10.1007/978-3-031-64159-6_7

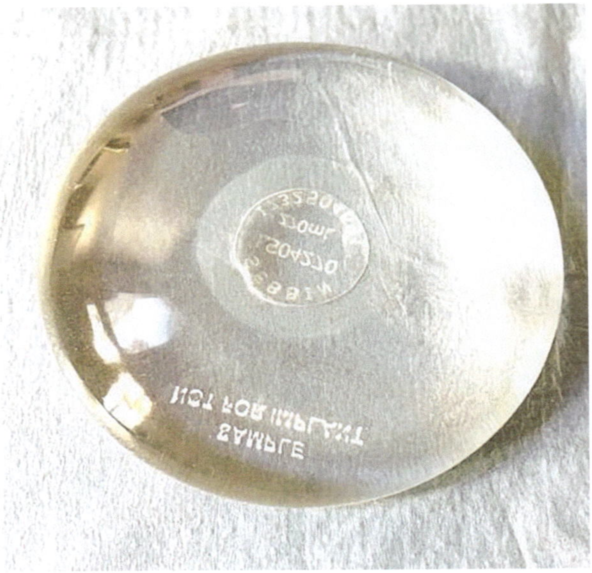

Fig. 7.1 Buttock implant

7.1.2 Imaging Protocol

Currently, there is no universally agreed-upon protocol or frequency for imaging in this context.

An ultrasound or an MRI is performed in case of suspicion of complication, or systematically for surveillance, usually after 5 years.

X-rays are not suitable for these locations.

7.1.3 Imaging Appearances

- **The ultrasound** is performed with the same high-frequency probe that for the breast and with the same program, adjusting the focal length and depth (Fig. 7.2a).
- **MRI** is performed in T2 STIR and WATER STIR "silicone only" sequences to differentiate the various components, physiological saline, or silicone [7]. This typically requires two to three planes of acquisition, most commonly in the axial and coronal orientations (Figs. 7.2b,c).
- **Importantly, no gadolinium contrast is administered during these MRI procedures.**
- The semiology of normal aspects and complications is the same as for breast implants, in ultrasound or MRI. The radiologist familiar with the semiology of breast implants can therefore easily interpret this type of examination.

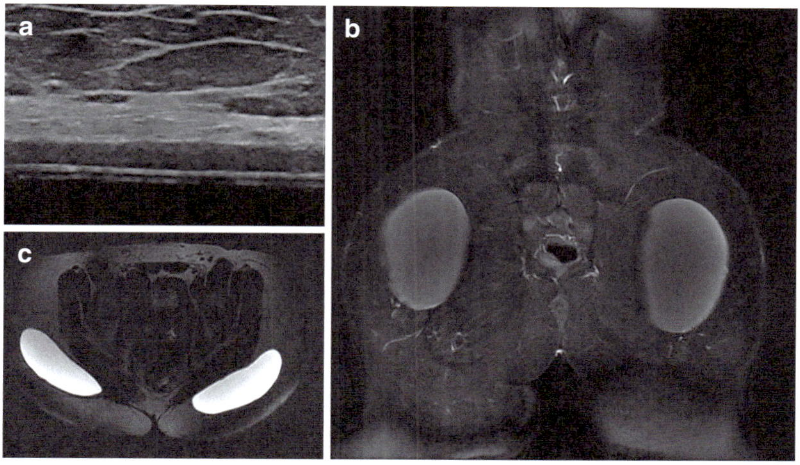

Fig. 7.2 Silicone-filled buttock implants. (**a**) Ultrasound image of the left buttock. (**b**) Pelvic MRI in coronal T2 STIR sequence, (**c**) Pelvic MRI in axial WATER STIR "silicone only" sequence. Intact silicone filled buttock implants within the thickness of the gluteus maximus muscle. In ultrasound, the capsulo-membranous complex and the anechoic aspect of the implant are like those of a breast implant. In MRI, the semiology is also the same as for a breast implant

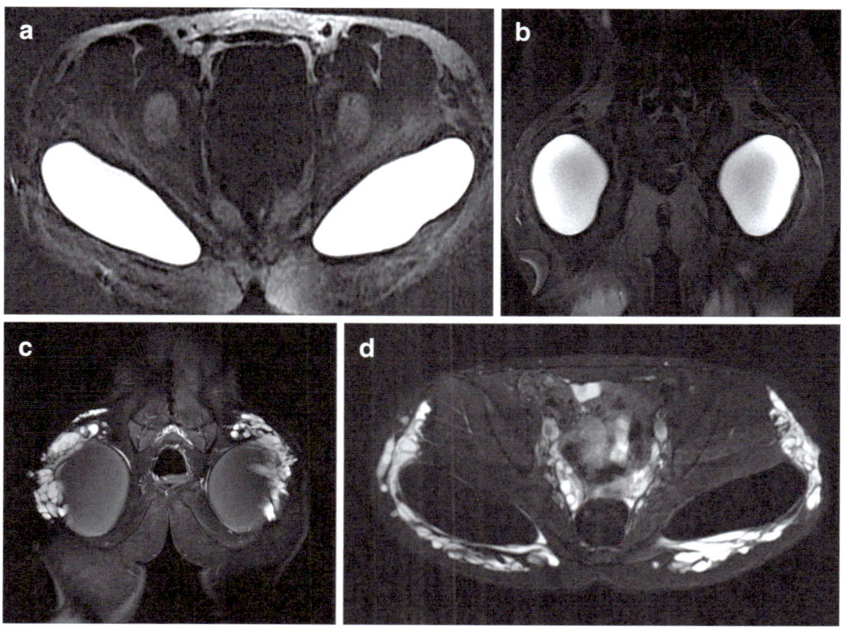

Fig. 7.3 MRI of the pelvis. Silicone filled Buttock implants associated with a free injection of hyaluronic acid. (**a**, **b**) axial and coronal WATER STIR "silicone only" sequences. (**c**, **d**): coronal and axial T2 STIR sequence (fat saturation). The silicone of the implants appears in hypersignal on the WATER STIR sequence "silicone only", while the injected hyaluronic acid around appears in hypersignal in T2 STIR sequence

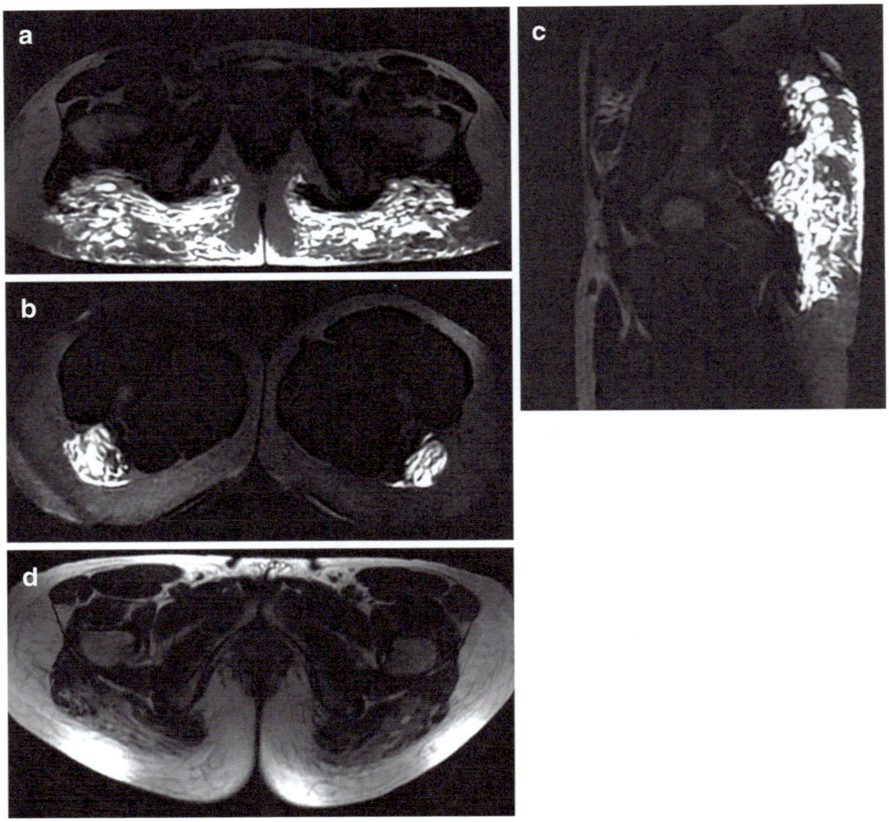

Fig. 7.4 Pelvic MRI. Free silicone intragluteal injection. (**a**, **b**) Axial WATER STIR "silicone only" sequence. (**c**) Sagittal WATER-STIR sequence on the left buttock. (**d**) Axial T2 without fat signal saturation. Free silicone intragluteal injection. The MRI confirms the silicone nature of the filling product and allows assessment of its distribution before a possible intervention. No fat necrosis is noted on this examination

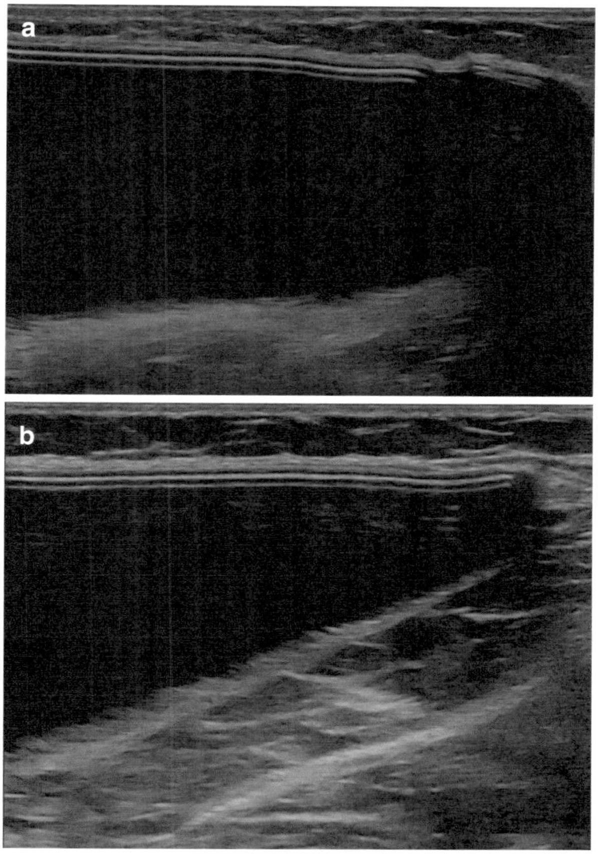

Fig. 7.5 Calf implants. (**a**) left ultrasound image, and (**b**) right ultrasound image. Normal saline implants put in place for aesthetic purposes to increase the curve. MRI is not indicated

7.2 Implants for Correction of Pectus Excavatum

Pectus excavatum is a congenital chest deformity characterized by a depression of the sternum, either medially or laterally. It affects about 1% of the population and represents 90% of chest wall deformities.

The most accepted cause is an abnormal length of the costal cartilages due to their hypergrowth. The deformation mainly affects the lower cartilages (from the third to the 7th).

7.2.1 Surgical Techniques

The deformity, primarily a cosmetic concern, can also lead to psychological distress and, in severe cases, cardiorespiratory issues. In younger individuals, conservative methods like the suction bell are highly effective. This device, worn for a few hours daily over several months, can help correct the deformity.

In adolescents, surgical options are available. The **Nuss procedure**, a minimally invasive thoracoscopic technique, involves inserting one or two bars inside the rib cage, secured with stabilizers, to reshape the chest. This method yields satisfactory outcomes [8, 9].

For less pronounced cases of pectus excavatum, **implant surgery** offers a solution primarily from an aesthetic perspective. It is considered a reference technique due to its simplicity, reliability, and minimal invasiveness. However, it's important to note that this approach is not designed to address any underlying cardiac or respiratory functional issue [10, 11].

7.2.2 Imaging Protocol and Appearances

Imaging is instrumental in designing custom implants that are easily placed under the pectoral muscles and tailored to each patient's unique anatomy. Preoperative chest CT scan is essential for calculating the Haller index (the ratio of the transverse diameter of the chest to the anteroposterior diameter between the sternum and vertebral body) (Fig. 7.6). This scan also measures the angle and height of the pectus deformity, aiding in the creation of a personalized implant.

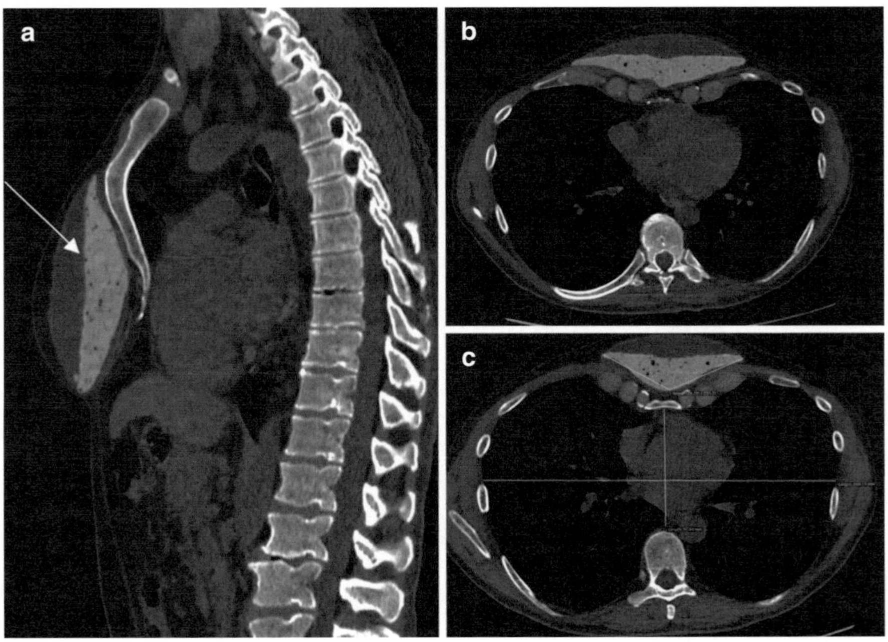

Fig. 7.6 Chest CT scan without contrast. Implant for pectus excavatum correction. Sagittal (**a**) and axial (**b**, **c**) sections. The CT scan serves a dual purpose: first, to assess the existing implant, which is visibly heterogeneous and deteriorated with peri-prosthetic effusion. Second, it facilitates various measurements and angle calculations, crucial for evaluating the severity of the deformity and determining the dimensions of a new, tailor-made implant for replacement

In cases where there's a suspicion of implant-related complications, an ultrasound or MRI can be conducted. The imaging characteristics are similar to those observed with breast implants.

References

1. Andrade GA, et al. Gluteal augmentation with silicone implants: a new proposal for intramuscular dissection. Aesth Plast Surg. 2017;41(4):872–7.
2. Frank SJ, et al. Aesthetic surgery of the buttocks: imaging appearance. Skeletal Radiol. 2014;43(2):133–9.
3. Lupon E, et al. Correction of calf atrophy with a custom-made silicone implant for reconstruction: an update. Aesthet Surg J. 2021;41(5):nP243–4.
4. Nguyen TT, Kilaru P. Plastic surgery and cosmetic procedures: augmentation and reconstruction procedures. FP Essent. 2020;497:27–36.
5. Chavoin JP, et al. Correcting of calf atrophy with a custom-made silicone implant: contribution of three-dimensional computer-aided design reconstruction: a pilot study. Aesthet Surg J. 2021;41(2):nP12–22.
6. Andjelkov K, et al. Safe composite calf augmentation: a staged procedure. Aesthet Surg J. 2021;41(2):nP26–35.
7. Niasme E, et al. Quantitative magnetic resonance imaging: differentiating soft tissue implants and fillers used in cosmetic and reconstructive surgery. Skeletal Radiol. 2021;50(1):231–7.
8. Torre M, et al. Blood metal levels after minimally invasive repair of pectus excavatum. Interact Cardiovasc Thorac Surg. 2021;33:76.
9. Cierpikowski P, et al. Surgical correction of pectus excavatum by the nuss procedure: a 15-year experience study. Adv Exp Med Biol. 2018;1047:31–40.
10. Chavoin JP, et al. The role of computer-aided design implant insertion in revision pectus surgery revision pectus surgery with implants. Ann Thorac Surg. 2021;112:e387.
11. Caro C, et al. Simultaneous correction of a pectus excavatum with tubular breast deformity using a custommade silicone implant. Arch Gynecol Obstet. 2021;303(4):1025–37.

Index

S. Cohen-Zarade, *Imaging of Plastic Surgery of the Breast and Other Implants*, https://doi.org/10.1007/978-3-031-64159-6

MIX
Papier aus verantwortungsvollen Quellen
Paper from responsible sources
FSC® C105338

If you have any concerns about our products,
you can contact us on
ProductSafety@springernature.com

In case Publisher is established outside the EU,
the EU authorized representative is:
Springer Nature Customer Service Center GmbH
Europaplatz 3, 69115 Heidelberg, Germany

Printed by Libri Plureos GmbH
in Hamburg, Germany